PENGUIN BOOKS

Gillian McKeith's Boot Camp Diet

Gillian McKeith is an internationally acclaimed holistic nutritionist. She presented *You Are What You Eat*, the hit Celador primetime television programme for Channel 4. She is also the author of the bestselling *You Are What You Eat*, the *You Are What You Eat Cookbook*, *Dr Gillian McKeith's Ultimate Health Plan*, *Dr Gillian McKeith's Shopping Guide*, *Gillian McKeith's Wedding Countdown Diet* and *Gillian McKeith's Food Bible*, all of which are published by Penguin.

Gillian McKeith's

BOOT CAMP DIET

FOURTEEN DAYS TO A NEW YOU!

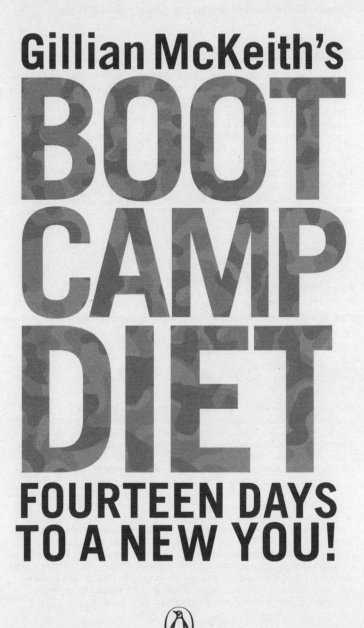

PENGUIN BOOKS

This book is dedicated to my lovely daughters

PENGUIN BOOKS

Published by the Penguin Group

Penguin Books Ltd, 80 Strand, London WC2R 0RL, England

Penguin Group (USA) Inc., 375 Hudson Street, New York, New York 10014, USA

Penguin Group (Canada), 90 Eglinton Avenue East, Suite 700, Toronto, Ontario,
Canada M4P 2Y3 (a division of Pearson Penguin Canada Inc.)

Penguin Ireland, 25 St Stephen's Green, Dublin 2, Ireland
(a division of Penguin Books Ltd)

Penguin Group (Australia), 250 Camberwell Road, Camberwell,
Victoria 3124, Australia (a division of Pearson Australia Group Pty Ltd)

Penguin Books India Pvt Ltd, 11 Community Centre,
Panchsheel Park, New Delhi – 110 017, India

Penguin Group (NZ), 67 Apollo Drive, Rosedale, North Shore 0632,
New Zealand (a division of Pearson New Zealand Ltd)

Penguin Books (South Africa) (Pty) Ltd, 24 Sturdee Avenue,
Rosebank, Johannesburg 2196, South Africa

Penguin Books Ltd, Registered Offices: 80 Strand, London,
WC2R 0RL, England

www.penguin.com

First published 2009
1

Set in New Clarendon
Designed by Smith & Gilmour, London
Printed in England by Clays Ltd, St Ives plc

ISBN: 978–0–141–03716–5

Every effort has been made to ensure that the information in this book is
accurate. The information in this book will be relevant to the majority of
people but may not be applicable in each individual case, so it is advised that
professional medical advice is obtained for specific information on personal
health matters and before embarking on any exercise programme. Neither the
publisher nor the author accepts any legal responsibility for any personal injury
or other damage or loss arising from the use or misuse of the information and
advice in this book. All vitamin, mineral and herbal supplements are sold in
varying strengths, so always check the dosage on the packaging.

www.greenpenguin.co.uk

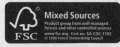

CONTENTS

BOOT CAMP

LEVEL ONE

DAY 1 ORIENTATION DAY

WELCOME TO YOUR FIRST DAY AT BOOT CAMP!

If it's weight you want to lose, you've come to the right place. That's the purpose of my Boot Camp, and the reason you and I are together. You are guaranteed to lose weight if you do what I tell you. As long as you follow exactly what I say, to the letter, you will succeed. And it will be easy and simple.

My Boot Camp gets results with weight loss. Millions of people around the world have witnessed first-hand on the telly how my overweight clients have lost enormous amounts of excess weight using my Boot Camp method.

But my philosophy is such that I don't want you fixated on your actual weight. As I always say, *'Weight is not so important, but your health is everything.'* Therefore there is no need to concentrate on 'losing weight' or 'gaining weight': aim instead to 'eat healthily', and the weight will take care of itself.

I am here to tell you that it's time to take back the reins of your body and life. You have more power within you than you probably realize to make a positive shift in your overall health, never mind just your weight.

BOOT CAMP PHILOSOPHY

My Boot Camp is a full-on, focused way of making positive changes. It lasts a short time, just 14 days, but has long-term results.

An important note: this is *not* to be confused with a crash diet. Crash diets ask you to adopt bad food habits in order to get very temporary results. My Boot Camp demands you adopt good food and lifestyle habits. And the results are anything but temporary.

My Boot Camp has been tried and tested on my own clients. I know it gets results and I want to pass those on to you. The words Boot Camp might sound daunting, but by committing yourself for 14 days, the habits will become ingrained and easy to follow for the next few weeks – and for the rest of your life. It gives you a foundation for healthy, happy living. Who wouldn't want that?

GETTING STARTED

You might think I am asking you to do a lot on this first day, but today we set the stage for the whole of my Boot Camp. It does get easier, and you will see and feel the changes in your body rapidly. So please do everything I ask of you, to the letter. It's best to start Day 1 on a weekend, or on your day off, as there is a lot to do in order to set a strong foundation.

Remember, there's good reason why I call it *Gillian's Boot Camp*. Boot Camp is known to be fast, furious, maybe even fun at times, and very results-driven. It starts out with a flurry but then gets easier. And my Boot Camp, unlike the military one, doesn't hurt in the least. So no excuses, please.

At the end, you will delight in the new you. You are now officially a rookie Boot Camper. So get on with your tasks right now. We have a lot to achieve. That's an order, and it's given with love!

The one thing you need right now is a notebook ...

TASK 1: DECLARATION OF INTENT

Open up your notebook, which I like to call your **Log Book**, and on the very first page I want you to write your **Declaration of Intent** (see page 216).

The **Declaration of Intent** is your most important first step. Take your time and think very carefully about what you 'want' to get out of Boot Camp. Then write it down on the Declaration form. This statement becomes your **Declaration of Intent**. I am not going to put words into your mouth, but your main motivation is likely to be that you are here to shift excess pounds and lose some weight. So if that's the case, write it down. By putting your intention on paper, it's as if it is with you and already happening.

So you write, think and act as though it is *there* right now. For example, write the words:

'I lose weight' or 'I lose a dress size.'

Writing, thinking and feeling in the present tense strengthens the vibration significantly. It is as if the 'want' is taking place right now. You can even give thanks and feel gratitude, as if you have already received it.

When you construct and write down these desires, you may keep them general at this point, since we will be breaking them down more specifically later, on Day 3. Therefore, at this early stage on Day 1, you might just jot down a general desire for improved health, increased confidence, more energy, a happier mood, looking younger, better overall well-being. You decide.

TASK 2: PROGRESS TRACKING

You will use your **Log Book** for **Progress Tracking**. Answer the questions outlined here *before* you get started. This is a necessary step, to make a note of your feelings of well-being on all levels. How you feel physically, mentally, emotionally and energetically is an integral part of the process. I want you to rate how you feel *now*, by making observations about yourself. These same questions will be answered not just today, but on Day 14 when you graduate from Boot Camp.

It is critical that you are brutally honest with yourself. This is the way to get the most out of *Gillian's Boot Camp*. Your answers must be based on exactly where you are right now, not where you want to be. These questions will identify early on your areas of potential resistance when it comes to your weight or general health.

RATE YOURSELF

On a scale of 1–10 (where **1** is a pathetic score like 'I'm a mess, I can barely drag myself out of bed in the morning' and **10** is a perfect score like 'I'm the Bomb, I could run a marathon today since I have so much energy'):

01 What's your mood like? Are you happy, depressed, apathetic, full of life? ☐

02 How much energy do you have? Do you feel like you could take on a sumo wrestler, or do you feel like a limp dish-rag most days? ☐

03 How well do you sleep? ☐

04 How do you feel when you wake up? ☐

05 How stressed out are you? ☐

06 Do you like yourself? ☐

When you come back to these questions in 2 weeks, I promise that you will see an amazing difference.

IT'S ALL ABOUT YOU

On a separate page in your **Log Book**, I want you to explore your thoughts, memories and emotions around food, both positive and negative. Feel how you would like to see this relationship in the future. The more you recognize your feelings and allow yourself to take note, the more your healing process will activate. Don't brush your feelings under the carpet. Do the opposite. Face yourself head-on. I once read a slogan that said, *'What you resist will persist.'* Put another way: *'Face it and let it go.'*

In my more than 15 years of nutritional private practice with clients, I have found that emotional baggage creates the biggest block to health and happiness. It is facing your feelings head-on and opening up emotionally that will allow you to make the changes you so dearly want. Write down as much as you need to.

No holding back here.

To perform this exercise, I need you to find some quiet time in a space that is peaceful. Listen to your breath going in and out for a few minutes. Imagine that your breath is filling up your entire body from your feet to your legs, to your torso, your arms, neck and head. You need not do anything here, just listen to your breath as you inhale and exhale.

After a few minutes of breath-listening, start to make notes. Recognize the memories and look at what comes up head on. Pretend that you are *looking at yourself* from a slight distance rather than being totally immersed in what you may recall or feel. See anger, see upset, see sadness, see frustration, see whatever is there. When you see it (whatever 'it' may be), view it as a colour or a patch of grey mist or a cloud-like substance. Then you can let go of it and see it fly to the sky, far and away. Or you could simply throw it away in the dustbin. Some people may want to write down on a piece of paper what it looks like and feels like, then build a little bonfire outside and drop the paper into the burning fire.

To help you flesh out these thoughts, take a look at the following triggers that should help.

ARE YOU EATING YOUR FEELINGS?

The Present

What is your relationship like with food right now? Is it positive? Negative? What kind of food do you eat or serve in your house today? How do you treat your kids (if you have kids) when it comes to food? Are you emotionally attached to food? Do you eat rubbish food when you get upset, scared, depressed or sad? Do you comfort eat?

Are there any emotional markers in your life today that are significant? Any big emotional trigger that still causes hurt, pain or anger? If so, do you feel it is resolved or still unresolved? Or do you use food to bury your feelings? Do you eat your feelings with chocolate cakes, pastries and éclairs?

The Past

What do you feel when you think of your childhood, or of any time period before today? Were you overweight as a child, teenager or young adult? What was your relationship with food as a child? What kind of food was served in your house? Was food ever used to reward you? Or to punish you? How so? Was there a lack of or an abundance of food? What types of food? Do you have certain memories of food or food aromas associated with loved ones so you like to eat it a lot, as a result? Or not eat it at all?

What was it like at mealtimes when you were a kid? Did you eat around a table? Was the family calm and relaxed or tense at mealtimes? Were you told to eat everything on your plate? What happened as a child if you did not eat everything on your plate? When you were upset or if you hurt yourself, did an adult comfort you with food? Looking back, was there ever a time in your life when you remember a marking point when you may have started to eat badly?

I remember one client, a professional international singing star, who told me that she used to sing with her granny all the time when she was a little girl. Then one day the singing stopped. Her granny fell ill, ended up in hospital and passed away shortly thereafter. But from the day that Granny stopped singing with her, my client became a chocolate cake junkie. Chocolate cake was Granny's favourite. Once my client could recognize the correlation between the feelings about her granny and the chocolate cake, she was on her way to a new realization of herself and went on to become one of the most amazing vocalists in the world.

Also, in your **Log Book**, record the following information:

Weight

This is the one and only time you should weigh yourself from now until the end of Boot Camp. I am not a fan of scales, and it does not help you one bit to be jumping on and off them every 5 minutes. In fact, at the clinic I never even had scales! The first problem with weighing yourself is that weight fluctuates. Keep in mind that muscle weighs more than flab. And you will be building plenty of new muscle here.

As you shed the fat, you should increase your muscle tone, and thus your weight could increase at times as well. But it doesn't matter if you put on some weight in the area of muscle tone. What matters is that overall, your weight will reduce, your muscle tone will increase and your health will improve.

Measurements

Just for Day 1, please take the following measurements.

>> Waist, bust, hips, thighs
>> Dress size or trouser size
>> BMI : Divide your weight in kilos by the square of your height in metres.
For example: 55kg divided by 1.55^2 (2.4025) = **22.9**

Below 18.5 = underweight
18.5–24.9 = normal
25–29.9 = overweight
Over 30 = obese

You can add comments to your **Log Book** any time you like. Some results are easily measurable, like losing a dress size. 'Feeling better' is harder to quantify, but I will offer guidelines on how to do it. It helps to keep a record of your moods, emotions, concentration levels and energy reserves. This will give you the best indication of how you are doing.

TASK 3: GENERAL HEALTH PROFILE (GHP)

This short quiz will give you a pretty good idea of where you stand with your general health. So please be true to yourself with your answers. Answer **YES** or **NO** to each question, and keep a record of your score in your **Log Book**.

General health

01 Are you generally free from pain and inflammation? **(Y/N)**

02 Do you wake up without an alarm clock, feeling energetic and ready to start the day? **(Y/N)**

03 Are your energy and mood consistently good throughout the day? **(Y/N)**

04 Are you able to think clearly and focus on what you are doing? **(Y/N)**

05 Are you positive and happy about life in general? **(Y/N)**

Lifestyle

06 Do you do exercise that noticeably raises your heart rate at least 4 times a week? **(Y/N)**

07 Do you get outside in fresh air and daylight for at least half an hour every day? **(Y/N)**

08 Do you walk or cycle, if going out locally, rather than automatically going by car? **(Y/N)**

09 Do you avoid alcohol, cigarettes and recreational drugs? **(Y/N)**

10 Do you take time out to relax every day? **(Y/N)**

Weight

11 Are you happy with your weight? **(Y/N)**

12 Are you happy with your muscle tone? **(Y/N)**

13 Is your stomach more or less flat (no doughnut round the middle)? **(Y/N)**

14 Do you avoid going on fad diets and yo-yo dieting? **(Y/N)**

15 Are you free of cellulite and flab? **(Y/N)**

Eating habits

16 Do you eat at least 5 servings of fruit and vegetables a day? **(Y/N)**

17 Do you avoid foods that contain sugar, refined carbohydrates, additives and preservatives? **(Y/N)**

18 Do you eat nuts and/or seeds daily? **(Y/N)**

19 Do you drink 8 large glasses of water or herbal tea a day, or maybe some veggie juices? **(Y/N)**

20 Do you eat 6 times a day: breakfast, snack, lunch, snack, dinner, snack? **(Y/N)**

How to score
Count the number of times you answered **YES.** This will rate your score.

If you scored: **16–20**
Well done! You are top of the game already. But you still need to get with my Boot Camp and improve on any negatives. No slacking off, as you have tremendous potential. I am sure you can see the areas where improvement is needed, so please stay focused. Make notes in your **Log Book** of the steps you need to action.

10–15

Not so good. There's still more work to be done. Massive room for improvement. I want to see real effort. No half measures. Plan everything and stick to it. It will be so worth it.

0–9

You have come to the right place, and not before time. The good news is that at least you've found *Gillian's Boot Camp*. Thank goodness for small mercies. You can only do better. You may have some OK aspects to your diet and lifestyle, but we have our work cut out. Do everything I say to the letter and then some, or else!

TASK 4: SHOPPING

Check your diary and commit to a time when you will go shopping in the next day or so. Tomorrow you're going to draw up your first **Action Plan** and **Shopping List**.

Superfood of the day

Aduki beans

Your new best friend is my 'King Bean of Weight Loss', the aduki bean. This small reddish-brown bean has a delicious, peppery, sweet-and-sour flavour. Adukis act like sponges, soaking up excess bloat, damp and fat in the body.

Day 1 end-of-day checkpoint

Have you completed the following?

☐ Declaration of Intent

☐ Progress Tracking

☐ General Health Profile

☐ Shopping Plan

Well done for today. You are now on your way, Boot Camper. From this day forward get to bed at a decent time (10:30 p.m. or before). See you tomorrow.

DAY 2 ACTION PLANNING

It's Day 2 – and you are now thinking consciously about your aims and objectives for Boot Camp.

TASK 1: PRIORITY ACTIONS

Today you set your priorities. So use your **Log Book** to make notes and plan how you will tackle each one.

1 Eating Habits

Refer back to your **General Health Profile** in Day 1. Look at your answers on eating habits and see where you need to make changes and focus your priorities.

>> Eat 6 meals a day. That's breakfast, snack, lunch, snack, dinner, snack. No skipping meals. I'm not into restricting food intake.

>> Vary your meal plans; in other words, do not eat the same foods day in, day out. You may have been a food rut eater until now, all too often just going for what is most familiar. That all changes today.

>> Include some raw food with each meal.

>> Have the most amount of food earlier in the day. So it's breakfast like a queen, lunch like a king and dine like a pauper.

2 Lifestyle Habits

Look back at your **General Health Profile** again. This time, focus on the lifestyle section. Work out what you are going to do to move that bahookee of yours and when you're going to move it. To lose weight, you must get active. It's not enough to just fit in what I call 'Lifestyle Habits' once or twice a week. I want you to move that bod of yours as much as you can throughout the day. For the duration of Boot Camp, find time to do a minimum of one hour of **Lifestyle Habits** every day. I am not asking you to become a fitness fanatic, but sitting in front of a computer screen, driving a car everywhere and sleeping in at weekends are simply not part of my blueprint.

Plan **how** you will move, **commit** to it and **log** it.

I insist that you walk or do some sort of exercise *before* you eat. A 15-minute walk at lunchtime is a cinch to fit in. You will think better; your mood will be happier; you will feel healthier.

You can also:

>> Walk to work, or park the car a few extra streets from the office.

>> If you are already physical, with a regular routine, expand that to take up a completely new activity or include new and different exercises. How about yoga, pilates, bicycling, chi gung, tai chi, stretching, kick-boxing, trampolining?

>> Get up 10 minutes earlier than normal and do some stretches or walk up and down the stairs (step on the spot if you don't have stairs) a few times.

>> Go out dancing, take up swimming, skip with a rope, visit the gym, play squash, take the stairs, go running, race the kids to the park, wash the car, vacuum the stairs with attitude, put some serious elbow grease into the housework!

Get on your bike to go to the shops for the groceries. Get the idea?

>> Most evenings I take my two wee daughters into the living room, turn up the CD player and we all dance like mad. It's fun; we sweat, and we all are happier afterwards for doing it.

3 Clear Out

Good riddance to bad rubbish. Get rid of the following during Boot Camp.

>> Table salt
>> Refined white sugar
>> Processed meats
>> Pizzas
>> Carbonated drinks
>> The white stuff (white bread, white pasta, white rice)
>> Cakes and biscuits
>> Crisps
>> Packaged foods with added sugar and table salts
>> Cow's milk
>> Cream
>> Black tea and coffee
>> Booze (c'mon, what did you expect? It causes cellulite anyway, and you don't want any more of that)
>> Hard cheeses
>> Chocolate (expect for raw cacao)
>> Sweets
>> Ice cream
>> Margarine
>> Butter
>> Wheat products

And before you start groaning that there's nothing left to eat, know this: you are going to eat more foods than you thought imaginable. You don't have to dump the entire list for ever. But you are in my Boot Camp, and as long as you are here, I demand full compliance. You want results and a fresh start. So get with the plan, on the double, and you will achieve exactly what you want and then some.

ABUNDANCE FOOD LIST

Leafy Green Vegetables

. . . .

Beet greens	Mustard greens
Chicory	Turnip greens
Collards	Parsley
Dandelion greens	Rocket
Endive	Romaine
Escarole	Sorrel
Iceberg lettuce	Spinach
Kale	Swiss chard
Loose-leaf lettuce	Watercress

Vegetables

. . . .

Artichoke	Chinese cabbage
Asparagus	Carrots
Aubergine	Cauliflower
Avocado	Celeriac
Beets	Celery
Broccoli	Courgettes
Brussels sprouts	Daikon

Green peas
Kohlrabi
Okra
Onions
Parsley
Parsnips
Peppers

Pok choi
Potatoes
Radish
Squash
Tomatoes
Turnips

Nuts

· ·

Almonds
Brazil nuts
Cashews
Filberts
Hazelnuts

Chestnuts
 Pecans
Pine nuts
Pistachios
Walnuts

Seeds

· ·

Chia seeds
Flax seeds
Shelled hemp seeds

Pumpkin seeds
Sesame seeds
Sunflower seeds

Flours

· ·

Amaranth
Hemp
Millet
Oat
Potato

Soya
Spelt
Sunflower seed
Tapioca

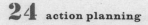

Sea Vegetables

Agar
Arame
Dulse
Hijiki
Kelp

Kombu
Nori
Sea palm
Wakame

Grains

Amaranth
Barley
Basmati rice
Buckwheat
Bulgar wheat
Corn

Kamut
Millet
Oats
Quinoa
Rye
Spelt

Beans

Aduki
Anasazi
Black turtle
Fava (broad beans)
Garbanzo
Great Northern

Lentils
Lima (butter beans)
Mung
Navy
Pinto
Soya

Fresh Herbs and Spices

Basil
Bay

Cardamom
Chervil

Cinnamon

Marjoram

Cloves

Mint

Coriander

Oregano

Cumin

Rosemary

Dill

Saffron

Fennel

Tarragon

Fenugreek

Thyme

Ginger

Herbal Teas

· ·

Chamomile

Melissa

Dandelion

Nettle

Fennel

Pau d'arco

Ginger

Peppermint

Ginseng

Red clover

Hawthorn

Rose hips

Horsetail

Slippery elm

Lemon balm

Spearmint

Liquorice

Valerian root

Fruit

· ·

Apples

Cranberries

Apricots

Currants

Bananas

Dates

Blackberries

Figs

Blueberries

Gooseberries

Cactus fruit

Grapes

Cherries

Guavas

Grapefruit

Huckleberries

Kiwi fruits

Kumquats

Lemons

Limes

Loganberries

Loquats

Lychees

Mangoes

Melons (banana, cantaloupe, honeydew, watermelons)

Mulberries

Nectarines

Papayas

Passion fruit

Peaches

Pears

Pineapple

Pomegranates

Strawberries

Umeboshi plums

Dried Fruit, but make sure that it is free of sulphur dioxide.

Other Foods

. . . .

Tofu

Tempeh

Fish

White meats

TASK 2: CHOOSE RECIPES

Go to my recipe section on page 141 and, along with the list above, plan your meals for the next few days. Use my **Meal Planner** on page 220 to get you started. My guide to an ideal day's intake (page 29) will give you an excellent framework to work with while you get everything in place.

TASK 3: SHOPPING LIST

If you haven't done a basic shop yet, get yourself down to the shops as soon as you can fit it in – even if you can only get a few of the ingredients. You've got to do this within the next 48 hours (allowing for busy schedules), if not sooner, so that by Day 4, and no later, you're eating fully in accordance with my Boot Camp.

Check your cupboards for food supplies. When you shop, get snack foods and include herbs and spices – buy them fresh, and include one or two herbal teas. Watch which aisles you go down at the supermarket. If the crisp aisle is calling out your name, take a wide berth and get yourself pronto to the fruit section. Don't let any 'Clear Out' items sneak into your basket.

TASK 4: FOOD DIARY

Write down everything you eat and drink, including the times, in your **Food Diary** sheets (see pages 219, 224, 228, 231, 234, 237, 239, 241, 242, 245, 247 and 248). These sheets must include every single morsel of food or drop of liquid that passes your lips. And I mean everything. No point in telling porky pies to yourself. So let's agree that it will be only the God's honest truth.

Last but not least, note how you feel before and after eating a meal, a snack and any food or beverage. Are you sleepy or tired, in a good or bad mood, itchy, headachy, full of mucus or just fine, more energized? Do you see or feel any physical changes?

Don't go looking for something that is not there. Simply take note of a physical feeling or emotion. You may not experience any change, and that's OK too. The end result

BOOTCAMP DIET
AN IDEAL DAY'S INTAKE

First thing:
Warm water with a
squeeze of lemon juice.

Breakfast smoothie:
1 banana, a cup of
strawberries and a cup
of blueberries.

Snack:
Hummus with carrot
and cucumber sticks.

Lunch:
Salad of mixed sprouts,
rocket, cherry tomatoes
and avocado with a lemon
and olive oil dressing.

Snack:
Carrot, beetroot and celery
juice with ginger (juice 2
carrots, 1 small beetroot,
2 stalks of celery and a
piece of root ginger).

Dinner:
Lemon sole with mangetout,
broccoli and kale.

Snack:
A small handful of almonds.

Drink:
2 litres of water over the day,
plus herbal teas such as
nettle, fennel, peppermint
and lemon balm.

is that you make conscious choices about food and lifestyle
as opposed to automated, mindless habitual reactions. So to
be clear: from the second you get up to the minute you go to
bed, document everything during Boot Camp.

Superfood of the day

Nettle tea
Nettles are one of the best energy pick-me-ups. They are rich
in iron and minerals, and are an essential part of my weight-
loss plans, as they keep you regular and help you get rid of
excess bloat. Drink 2–3 cups daily.

Day 2 end-of-day checkpoint

Have you …

☐ Drawn up your shopping list?

☐ Scheduled a time to go shopping for the ingredients?

☐ Looked over your Priority Actions?

☐ Planned the best time to fit in some physical activity?

☐ Started your Food Diary?

Get shopping. Find your kitchen, start cooking and have a great day. You are off to a fabulous start.

DAY 3 GOALS

Welcome to Day 3. How are you feeling? Organized, I'll bet, now you've planned your menus and been shopping. Doesn't it feel great?

What I have in store for you today is goal-setting. There's no point signing up for a Boot Camp without knowing what you hope to achieve. And nobody knows that better than YOU.

Why do I want you to set goals? Because, frankly, they're one of the most powerful tools there is when it comes to getting what you want in life. They expand, grow and strengthen the energy of success. Ask any high achiever how they got where they are, and they'll tell you they knew exactly where they were headed and by which route.

The good news here is that you are already on your way. By joining *Gillian's Boot Camp*, you are now on the path! Remember your **Declaration of Intent**? That's your overall Primary Objective – what you're going to have achieved in three months' time. Today we set the goals that will allow you to achieve your Primary Objective. Your goals should be positive, achievable and motivating. And you need to visualize them as if they've already happened. I'm telling you, it's easy and fun. Just follow through with me. Here's all you need to do:

TASK 1: SETTING YOUR GOALS

Use your **Log Book** and see my **Goal Setting Sheet** on page 222 to get you started.

WORK OUT HOW TO GET THERE

It's important that your goals are achievable and manageable, so think about what steps it will take for you to achieve your Primary Objective, and break it down into an Action Plan such as Step 1, Step 2, Step 3 and so forth.

For instance, if you want more energy, your first step might be to get more sleep. Your second might be to cut down on stimulants such as caffeine, alcohol and sugar. And then you might want to do more exercise, a guaranteed energy-booster. Write down the actual steps you intend to action underneath your Primary Objective. This is the way to ensure your success on all levels.

Example:

Objective: I feel energetic

Goal 1: Be in bed by 10:30 p.m.

Goal 2: Cut down on stimulants.

Goal 3: Take 30 minutes' exercise a day.

YOU THE ARTIST

You are the creator and the artist of your own life. So now I want you to draw your **Primary Objective** as a picture. You don't have to be a great artist – everyone can draw. We can all create. Sketch yourself having achieved your goal, therefore looking slim, doing something energetic – whatever your goal is.

If you're feeling really creative, you may also like to sketch some of your interim goals towards your objective – a comic strip of the next few weeks or months, for example.

Repeat this process for all your goals, each on a new sheet of paper within your **Log Book**. Your thoughts have powerful energy and this energy only increases when you write it down; even more so when you draw the pictures. When you write and draw and create real physical pictures of your goals, your original thoughts become actions in their own right. Your thoughts, your words and your actions have great power to action your dreams. You are far more powerful than you know. Nothing is outside your grasp. The power is within you to achieve everything you desire in your health and in your life, so reach for the stars!

TASK 2: DAILY MINI-GOALS

Now that you have your Primary Objective in place, you can pick out the **Mini-Goals** that you achieve day by day over the first part of Boot Camp. I'm talking about the little goals – trying a new food, going for a swim, or shopping at the health food store!

Write your **Daily Mini-Goals** into your **Log Book**. As soon as you achieve one, tick it off – a big, bold tick, or a star (a gold one if you like).

REWARDS

A great way to keep yourself motivated on those more challenging days is to promise yourself rewards. Of course, I don't mean ice creams or takeaways! Get imaginative and think of healthy treats you'll look forward to. Start a list in your **Log Book**. Examples of rewards for meeting your daily goals could be:

>> A bowl of delicious berries
>> A hot bath with essential oils
>> An hour of me-time to read a novel

Then, for bigger goals:

>> A massage
>> A manicure
>> A trip to the theatre

THE SATISFACTION SCALE

This is a handy guide I've developed to help you get in touch with
your TRUE hunger. No more eyes that are bigger than your belly!
It takes a bit of practice, but the rules are easy: **Eat at level 1 and
stop at level 4.**

LEVEL	HOW YOU FEEL	WHAT TO DO
EMPTY	Your stomach is uncomfortably empty. You're starving.	Always eat BEFORE you reach this level.
01	Your stomach's empty, there's a sensation of hunger.	It's time to eat. Drink something BEFORE you eat rather than during. Follow with raw fruit or salad.
02	A pleasant feeling – you're either eating slowly and comfortably, or have just eaten and are digesting.	Keep eating slowly. Take time to digest.
03	You start to feel satisfied.	Chew until your food becomes liquid. Connect with the food and enjoy it. Notice impending satisfaction.
04	The point of optimum comfort. You feel satisfied – no hunger or discomfort.	Stop – even if there is food on your plate or another course on the menu! You will not be sent to your room!
FULL	Now you're uncomfortable. Your abdomen swells. You may feel stuffed to the gills and nauseous.	Stop. Rest or go for a stroll, breathe deeply. Reflect on what made you eat too much. Commit to stopping at Level 4 next time.

And, for when you finish this Boot Camp:

>> A holiday
>> A new outfit
>> A meal in a fashionable restaurant

Superfood of the day

Parsley
I call parsley the culinary multivitamin, as it is so nutrient-dense. Great for balancing blood sugar levels, oedema and bloating. And it's available everywhere, so no excuses that you can't find it! 2–3 times weekly is fine.

Day 3 end-of-day checkpoint

Have you …

☐ Written down your Primary Goal and the steps required to get you there, and sketched yourself having achieved them?

☐ Written your Daily Mini-Goals in your Log Book?

☐ Started thinking of some rewards?

☐ Familiarized yourself with the Satisfaction Scale?

With these principles under your belt, you can garner the best results. You now have a clear picture of where you are going. Stay focused.

DAY 4 TIME MANAGEMENT

Welcome to Day 4. Are you coping well with your tasks so far? Or do you wish there were more hours in the day? Well, today's the day you and I help create them!

I'm no stranger to feeling time-starved. That's exactly why I've devised my Boot Camp, with busy, multi-tasking people like you in mind. Yes, there are huge demands on our time nowadays. But it *is* possible to manage family, work, friends, interests, chores, errands, shopping, exercise (yes, even the last one!).

I'm going to teach you a skill that will make the following days and months – even the rest of your life – easier: Time Management.

The main goal of Time Management? Finding more time to look after YOURSELF. Not freeing up hours so you can spend them chained to your desk. Not realizing you have more time to clean the loo or iron your kids' clothes. I'm talking about restructuring your days so that you have more time to exercise, enjoy your meals, have quiet time for you. I want to help you to have a better quality of life.

TASK 1: WORK OUT WHERE YOUR TIME IS GOING

In your **Log Book** create a table for writing down everything you do today. I know it seems laborious, but it will pay off.

In the first column, note the action, however small. I want EVERYTHING recorded (it'll be a long list!). In the second column, say why you did it – was it because you wanted to, had to, or another reason? In the third column, note the time this took. **I've filled in the first three rows as an example.**

WHAT I DID	WHY I DID IT	TIME IT TOOK
Made breakfast for the family	I had to	15 mins
Read the newspaper	I wanted to	10 mins
Chatted to my neighbour	I couldn't get away from her!	25 mins

If you look at the middle column, you'll find your precious time is used up in three ways:

01 Things you HAVE to do, such as preparing meals, going to work (or at least you have decided that you *'have to'*. The truth is that in life you don't actually *'have to'* do anything, unless you decide that it's important to you).

02 Things you CHOOSE to do, such as watching TV, reading. This is where most people feel time-starved.

03 Things you DON'T HAVE TO DO but you do them anyway because you think you should or ought to, such as running errands as favours, attending social events because you feel obliged, rather than want to – even having conversations! (Note: Once you get in touch with how you feel at the core of your body, and not just in the thoughts in your head, you will be more sensitive to what really feels right to you, in other words, what really matters to you.)

Go through your list with three different-coloured highlighter pens, dividing what you did into these categories. You'll notice they can encroach on each other. Maybe you think you HAVE to do something, but on reflection it wasn't that essential? If you didn't do everything in the 'HAVE to' category, would the world end? Well, no, but family life for example is nicer if you all eat breakfast together, so maybe, in fact, you CHOOSE to do the breakfast thing. It's empowering to feel they are your CHOICES. When you can calm the mind and feel your body at gut level, you can start to make contact with who you really are and what you really want.

The third category is tricky. If you're a helpful person, or simply find it difficult to say no, doing things for others can be a real time thief. Whether it's unwanted sales calls, a friend needing a hand, or the boss assuming you want overtime, this group needs working on! If you say 'no' to people kindly and politely, they rarely object (*I'd love to come over, but I'm very busy this evening, sorry*).

You then need to figure out why it's taking you so long to do the things you HAVE to do. Here's a clue: procrastination.

TASK 2: LEARN TO TAKE ACTION AND STOP PROCRASTINATING

That means no more wasting time.

If you often find yourself immersed in all manner of projects that aren't helping you achieve what you actually need to, you're procrastinating. Maybe you're tidying rooms that don't really need to be tidied, because you're putting off a difficult phone call. A friend of mine is a student, and whenever she's on a tight deadline, she told me she finds herself doing chores she'd never normally dream of, such as cleaning out cupboards or de-scaling the kettle – all just an effort to distract herself from her essays. Sound familiar?

The key to being more productive is working to a plan. So in your **Log Book**, find a fresh page and jot down a list of everything you must do today. Now, pick the item you most dread doing. This is the one you are absolutely, definitely going to do – the sooner the better.

TIPS ON ASSEMBLING MEALS IN MINUTES

01 Plan your meals in advance

02 Use canned beans and lentils without salt or sugar added. Rinse well

03 Alternatively, soak beans and lentils in plenty of water overnight to reduce cooking time. Lentils and mung beans cook at top speed once soaked

04 Good store-cupboard basics include olive oil, tamari soy sauce, lemons, miso, dried herbs, root ginger, canned beans, frozen peas, tofu, nuts, seeds, canned fish, canned water chestnuts and quick-cooking grains such as millet, quinoa, buckwheat and buckwheat noodles

05 Use sprouted lentils, pulses and beans. These can be eaten raw in salads, as snacks or added at the end of cooking to stir-fries, soups and casseroles for extra nutrition and texture. You can easily find sprouted seeds in health stores and supermarkets

06 Eat more raw food. You don't have to wait for it to cook

07 Cook the day before and then everything is ready when you come home, or do a big cook-off on a Sunday and freeze some for alternate days

Choose a positive affirmation (like a kind of mantra) to say to yourself whenever you find you're veering off course. It could be: 'Just do it!' 'Let's go!' Or, as another friend of mine likes to say, *'Eat that frog!'* (I've never really understood that, but I certainly wouldn't fancy eating a frog, so I can only guess she's referring to getting an unpleasant job over and done with.) Write your mantra on sticky notes and place them around your home and office. If anyone or anything distracts you and causes you to start procrastinating, silently repeat your mantra.

Here's the best bit. When the mantra works and you *do* just do it, you can treat yourself. Remember the list of rewards you compiled yesterday? Here's where it comes in handy. You may reward yourself now and every time you successfully use your mantra, take action and stop procrastinating. Well done! The more you manage your day and the less you procrastinate, the more hours you'll have free for YOU.

Superfood of the day

Flax/Linseeds

Flax seeds are packed with healthy fats which I call 'thinnies' to keep your weight down. 2–4 dessertspoons daily. Check out *roasted* flax seeds, as they are absolutely delicious and so crunchy!

Day 4 end-of-day checkpoint

Have you ...

☐ Filled out your time-management sheet?

☐ Worked out where your spare time is going?

☐ Committed to saying 'No' more often?

☐ Vowed to plan each day and write to-do lists?

☐ Chosen a mantra to stop yourself procrastinating?

☐ Rewarded yourself for achieving Task 2?

You have the tools to use your time in the most positive way. You can literally soar. Anything is possible. See you tomorrow, ready for action.

DAY 5 RESISTANCE IS FUTILE

Welcome to Day 5 – and well done for getting here. This tells me you're committed! Today's message: RESISTANCE IS FUTILE.

You've been a model Boot Camper so far, so don't let even an ounce of destructive inner talk sabotage your success.

I always say to my clients that *'what you resist will persist'*. So my goal here is to help you dissolve the resistance. At this point, you're probably thinking. *'What is she on about? Gillian's finally flipped.'* But after many years of experience with clients in private practice, plus working with TV show participants, I know all too well that now is the time when the 'Big R' for 'Resistance' might kick in.

You want to do well on my Boot Camp, of course. But many bad habits are ingrained, and the subconscious mind often likes to reinforce them. There's another shorter word for resistance: I call it 'EXCUSES'.

The following are the most common excuses I hear for not living healthily. Something here is bound to strike a chord:

01 'I'm too busy'

We talked about this yesterday, so you know I understand where you're coming from. Getting to grips with new ideas, foods, menus – adopting a new lifestyle – takes time. But you're busy. And before you know it, your finger is dialling the local takeaway joint or you are mindlessly stuffing a packet of cheesy crisps in your gob. But poor-quality food does not provide you with the energy and nourishment you need to cope with life's challenges. Healthy food does. That's the irony.

02 'I'm too stressed to do all this'

Good nutrition and exercise help you cope with stress. But when you've had a hard day, your subconscious might tell you that the last thing you need is a punishing health regime (which of course it is *not*!). Your subconscious then tells you that what you really need is half a bottle of white wine or a beer, or your usual coffee and cigarettes. Here's the secret: you're already punishing yourself with your mind and all that wasted judgement. All that stuff you make up in your mind stresses you and depletes you even more of energy. In other words, when you tell yourself these negative messages of resistance or excuses, it does not serve you and you only tire yourself out further. Escape the cycle of destruction now and give your body and mind a fighting chance to beat stress.

03 'Healthy food is too expensive'

Rubbish! I'm talking fresh, unprocessed, natural foods here. It is not so expensive. My foods, such as brown rice, quinoa, buckwheat groats, lentils, beans, fresh seasonal fruits and vegetables are all far cheaper than red meats, pork and packaged meals.

You can prepare delicious meals, bursting with nutrients, from the simplest, cheapest of ingredients. No one can persuade me that brown rice and beans cost the earth. They simply do not! My ears are closed to this sorry excuse because I've heard it all before, from the overweight takeaway-and-processed-white-bread junkies. *'I can't afford to eat healthily.'* So with that said, you can now toss out this excuse once and for all.

CHEAPER BY THE DOZEN

Check out my shopping lists and see for yourself (all prices listed were collected on 23 October 2008):

UNHEALTHY SHOPPING LIST

All-butter croissants x 6:	£1.98
Bottles of beer x 6:	£5.00
Cheese Strings:	£2.38
Choc ices x 8:	£1.99
Coco Pops:	£2.79
Crisps x 6:	£1.28
Double chocolate gateau:	£2.00
Family pork pie:	£2.69
Instant Coffee 100g:	£1.75
Margarine 250g:	£1.28
Pepperoni pizza:	£3.99
Sliced white bread:	£1.29
TOTAL:	**£28.42**

GILLIAN'S SHOPPING LIST

Bag of apples:	£1.68
Dried chickpeas:	£0.59
Fairtrade bananas x 7:	£1.29
Fresh mackerel:	£1.89
Herbal teas x 20:	£0.83
Organic brown rice:	£1.23
Organic carrots:	£0.96
Organic lettuce:	£1.09
Organic porridge oats:	£1.10
Red cabbage:	£1.03
Red split lentils:	£0.96
Sunflower seeds 200g:	£0.44
TOTAL:	**£13.09**

04 'My family won't eat THAT!'

So what? Does that mean you can't eat it either? On the contrary, you must first nourish and love yourself before you can love another. So take care of you. Granted it's easier to achieve most things in life when your loved ones are supporting you. But if your partner or your family don't care for your diet and insist on eating all the foods you're trying to leave behind, let them. It was your decision to join this Boot Camp. The benefits are yours for the taking. Once they see how happy, healthy, slim and fit you become, hopefully they'll soon get behind you. We can influence the people around us by being the example of change. We don't need to preach to or require acceptance from others in order to be whole and fulfilled. But you still must stand on your own two feet and be who you really are. So take a stand, and that, my friend, is an order.

TASK 1: NO MORE EXCUSES

Think about what excuse or excuses most ring true with you.

Write the overriding excuse in big bold letters at the top of a page in your **Log Book**. Underneath I want you to write a list of every single reason you can think of why this excuse, your resistance, is simply not justified. Please feel free to add some other, lesser excuses if you feel they are niggling at you.

Now turn your negative excuse into a positive statement. But make it realistic, too. It's an unrealistic big leap, for instance, to expect to go from *'I hate healthy food'* to *'I adore it'*. Therefore, find the middle ground. In other words, step it up one level higher.

So instead it would be more realistic and helpful to go from *'I hate healthy food'* to *'I'm open to trying healthier foods'*, or simply *'I'll try it'*. Other examples of stepping it up to a more positive statement could be: *'Healthy eating will help my stress'*; or *'I feel healthier or look better when I eat good food'*; or *'Making time for a healthier lifestyle pays off'*. I think you get the gist of the possibilities to make it work for you.

Write this new statement – this anti-excuse – in big bold letters across the bottom of your page.

This is your new voice. The excuse you wrote at the top of the page is your old, full-of-resistance voice. That voice is now history. I didn't say it's gone for ever; after all, history

SWITCH OFF YOUR NEGATIVE INNER TALK

Next time that inner voice creeps in, remember, you don't *have* to react to it. There are several things you can do. First, do something different. If you've had a stressful day or an argument with your partner and your inner voice is telling you a glass of wine or a tub of ice cream is the answer, do something to take your mind off it. Go for a walk, phone a friend, run a bath. Distract yourself.

If it persists, close your eyes and imagine two volume switches, side by side. As the voice starts to tell you what to do, see yourself reaching for the left-hand switch and turning it right down. Once you've muted your negative inner voice, reach for the right-hand switch and start to turn it up. Now you're turning up the volume on your positive voice, hearing your anti-excuse and all those reasons you wrote down why resistance is futile, growing louder and louder in your head. You see? You *can* control your thoughts *and* your actions.

Try this visualization trick every time resistance sets in. You'll soon have broken the pattern and set up healthier habits for life.

is always there to be told. But when you realize that you are engaging in that old negative history stuff, just take note and say, *'Oh, there's that old stuff I used to do, that's interesting, and now I let it go.'* You don't need that one any more. People think they can't change their old entrenched habits. Well, I'm here to tell you that you can change. Where I come from, there's an old Scottish saying: *'Nothing changes if nothing changes.'*

In other words, is your current way of thinking working for you? If your way is not serving your best interests, now is the prime time to change things, as we can embark upon a whole new path together.

TASK 2: CLUTTER CLEAR

Check around you: How cluttered are your surroundings? Is your kitchen clean and clear? Is your bedroom in order? When the house (and office and car and everything else around you) is tidy and organized, it's amazing how much easier it is to get yourself in order too. Take some time today to create clarity in your home, especially in the kitchen.

Superfood of the day

Seaweed

Seaweeds are bursting with essential minerals that aid weight loss. Need I say more? Make seaweed your best friend. Add seaweeds to soups, stews and salads, make avocado sushi, snack on spicy seaweed strips (from health food stores) and surprise yourself with my recipe for Mango and Pineapple Jelly on page 211.

Day 5 end-of-day checkpoint

Have you ...

☐ Picked the primary excuse or excuses that most cause you to resist change?

☐ Made a list of all the reasons your excuse is not valid?

☐ Chosen a more positive statement to change your way of thinking?

☐ Committed to 'do something different' whenever your negative inner voice kicks in?

☐ Tried the 'volume switch'?

Ditching negativity makes you feel lighter. From this day forward, Boot Campers, no more excuses to hold you back. You are well on your way now.

DAY 6
CHECKING IN WITH YOURSELF

Welcome to Day 6, Boot Camper! How are you doing?
Not sure? That's OK, because today we review what you've
been up to so far. We'll identify your strengths so you can
congratulate yourself; and take note of any areas of
weakness so you can work on them.

This is where your **Log Book** comes in handy. Pour
yourself a nice cup of herbal tea, sit down, and read through
everything you've recorded so far, for Days 1 to 5. Off you go.

Now, on a first reading, what are your impressions? Are you
doing well and enjoying the challenge of the Boot Camp?
Or has it been a struggle? Are you dealing with the areas
where you scored low in your **General Health Profile**?

TASK 1: PROGRESS CHECKLIST

To make this easier, jot down some answers to the following
series of questions. Feel free to use highlighter pens or
underline or write notes on any of the pages you've already
written on in your **Log Book**. It's *your* record of *your*
experience. It sometimes helps to find patterns if, for
example, you mark the page every time you've recorded a
negative thought – or every time you mention something
you've enjoyed.

01 What have you found easiest so far about the
Boot Camp?

02 What has seemed hardest?

03 What new foods have you most enjoyed?

04 Have you felt hungry or had cravings for certain foods at any point?

05 How have you felt before and after exercising?

06 Have you had any slips, and not stuck to the Boot Camp? If so, when, and why?

07 Have any of the tasks been particularly difficult for you?

08 Is your Log Book an honest recollection of how the past 5 days have been, or have you missed anything out?

09 When have you felt most sad or frustrated?

10 When have you felt your most happy and optimistic?

Finding patterns

I designed these questions to help you look for patterns in your experience of the Boot Camp so far, and identify where you may need to concentrate your efforts.

Did any patterns emerge for you?

Maybe you found that you tend to think about food and treats most at a certain point in the day? And this just might be the point at which your colleagues tend to offer round the biscuit tin at work? In which case, now that you've noted how this makes you feel, you can plan ahead. Next time, offer to run an errand as soon as you hear the rattle of the tin. Or find a convenient excuse to visit a department on another floor, till all danger has passed!

You may also have recognized more positive patterns. For example, take note of your moods around exercise. Maybe you're in the habit of dreading physical activity, but your **Log Book** has shown you that you always feel happier, more positive and energized after it. Remember this pattern and use it as an incentive next time you don't feel like going for that walk.

TASK 2: PERSONAL REPORT

Use the information you've gleaned from the task above to come up with your own personal Boot Camp progress report. I want you to write down the top three areas in which you're excelling, as an incentive to keep you on track. And then write down the three areas in which you're struggling, even if only a little, so you know to prioritize these as we move forward.

Here's an example of what you could write. I've filled it out for you, just to give you the sense of what I am talking about here and to help you out, but I expect you to do your own:

The Positives

01 I've stuck to my exercise plan and enjoyed it.

02 I always complete the tasks Gillian sets me.

03 I'm developing a taste for new foods. (Gillian says: Brilliant! Keep it up!)

The Areas to Work On

01 I'm struggling to quit caffeine.

02 I find it hard to say no when people offer me food.

03 I need to get to bed earlier. (Gillian says: Don't stress about it – identifying these issues is the first step to beating them)

Superfood of the day

Avocado

Avocados are a fantastic protein-rich snack food. Mash one up, or add to a smoothie to give it a creamy texture. Avocados contain healthy, good fats that can help keep you slim and trim as well as nourish metabolism. So, for goodness sake, don't avoid them. If you don't eat enough good healthy fats you can actually get fat and ill!

Day 6 end-of-day checkpoint

Have you …

☐ Read through your Log Book so far?

☐ Answered the questions on my Progress Checklist?

☐ Looked for Positive and Negative Patterns in your week?

☐ Identified your 3 Strongest and Weakest Areas?

☐ Checked how your typical day's Food Intake compares with my ideal?

See you tomorrow. You are doing great.

DAY 7
WHAT'S YOUR MOTIVATION?

Welcome to Day 7. You've been a Boot Camper for a whole week now. I'll bet it's been a life-changing week for you – in a good way, of course!

MOTIVATION

Motivation in bucketfuls is the aim today, to keep you going through the tricky times. Motivation is the drive to achieve your goal. Motivation can apply to any aspect of your life. Basically, there are two ideas in life that motivate us. The first is the desire to *get away* from something we don't want. The second is the desire to *reach for* something we really do want.

It might help to think of the 'carrot and stick' analogy. Are you chasing the carrot (positive) or fleeing from the stick (negative)?

The best motivation is always to think carrot, not stick. Keep your focus positive – on where you're headed, not where you've been. Let me give you some examples:

STICK

Feeling too knackered for sex.

CARROT

Having boundless energy and a healthy libido.

STICK

Being overweight and unfit.

CARROT

Being a healthy weight for your size and enjoying regular exercise.

STICK

Leaving your dead-end job.

CARROT

Being hired for a better-paid, more fulfilling role.

You see what I'm getting at? Carrots are the real positive motivating factors. These are going to get you through the tough times and move you towards your goals. Think **CARROT** every time. Got it?

TASK 1: DOWN WITH DEMOTIVATORS (THE SABOTAGERS)

I want you to identify those people who have a negative effect on your life: the demotivators (who I sometimes call 'the sabotagers'). We all know them, and almost everyone has at least one or more sabotager in his or her life; but we don't need to let them drag us down. I'm talking about those folk who are happy to remain undernourished, unmotivated, possibly overweight, unfit, unsupportive and have little or no spark for life. So maybe there are friends who don't appreciate your commitment to the Boot Camp and are always trying to lure you out to pubs and bars. Or family members who bemoan the new foods you bring home or object to you taking time out to exercise.

I'm not asking you to cut these people out of your life. I understand you may love and care for them. But I'm asking you to set some mental boundaries so that their negativity doesn't keep you down. I don't want them to sabotage your healthy way of living. They probably don't even know they're doing it – but on a subconscious level, the healthy new you might be a perceived threat to their persona or lifestyle. Stand your ground; establish your convictions in life and what's really important to you. Most important, get to know who you really are and move in the direction that serves you well.

In your **Log Book**, jot down some useful responses to use next time one of your demotivators tries to upset your plans. Remember, you don't need to apologize or make excuses, just be firm and be prepared. If they put up resistance, I find repetition soon gets the message across. So, here are some examples I would like you to repeat after me:

>> 'Thank you for the invitation, but I have other plans.'
>> 'I'd rather have this, thank you.'
>> 'No, thank you, I'm not hungry.'
>> 'If you don't like it, make your own!'

See – easy, wasn't it?

If you find you need to put some distance between you and some of your demotivators, a good solution is to seek out other people more like the new you (or rather more like the *real* you). See what clubs and classes are on offer in your area, where you'll meet like-minded exercisers, or people with interests and outlooks more like you. A client of mine has made a whole new group of friends since joining a running club. One colleague has joined a meditation group and attends every Wednesday evening. And another friend has become somewhat of a star on the local salsa scene!

KNOWLEDGE IS POWER

You're learning more about nutrition as every day passes. And this knowledge also acts as motivation. Knowing how bad junk food affects your body, your weight, your thought processes and your soul will motivate you not to choose it. Knowing how well a good, nourishing breakfast sets you up for the day motivates you to forgo the fry-up.

You'll probably find that during the course of Boot Camp you naturally gravitate towards more positive, inspiring people, and they to you. Your energy vibration shifts, and thus you may attract a different type of person and may subsequently be attracted to a different type of person as well. Make the most of it. Have fun! With new habits, new hobbies and new friends, not to mention my support, you have all the motivation and now the tools you need to succeed.

And what if you slip up one day? You might briefly lapse into an old habit or negative choice. So what? I say. Just take note of it. You can simply say, *'Hey, that's interesting'* – that's all you need to do. Then move on. Get over it. Most important, do not fret. Don't beat yourself up. Simply come on back into the next day's Boot Camp and carry on changing your life for the better!

Gillian's Quick Quiz

01 Which of the following contains omega-3 fatty acids to help shift those unwanted pounds?
a. A Cornish pasty
b. Bananas
c. A salmon steak

02 Which of the following does not contain caffeine?
a. Dandelion tea
b. Coffee
c. Cola

03 Which of these won't get your bowels moving if you're constipated?
a. Prunes
b. Nettle tea
c. White bread

04 Which of these is a good source of easy-to-digest protein?
a. Quinoa
b. Kebabs
c. Bacon

05 Which bean have I named as the Weight Loss Bean and one you should eat regularly for keeping that weight down?
a. Red kidney
b. Soya
c. Aduki

06 Which of the following fruit has the highest vitamin C content per 100g?

a. Oranges
b. Blackcurrants
c. Mangoes

07 Which of the following provides a good source of both the omega-3 and omega-6 essential fats?
a. Hemp
b. Olive oil
c. Avocados

08 Which of the following is a good source of calcium and magnesium needed for healthy bones and teeth?
a. Rice
b. Apples
c. Tahini

09 Which of the following is best for keeping blood sugar levels stable?
a. Baguette
b. Oats
c. Cornflakes

10 Which of the following can enhance liver detoxification and therefore be a weight-loss supporter?
a. White wine
b. Fish fingers
c. Grapefruit

Answers:
(**1**) c – Oily fish such as salmon, mackerel, trout are the best source of omega-3s. (**2**) a – Dandelion tea. It's also a fabulous addition to any weight-loss programme, due to its high mineral content and diuretic properties. (**3**) c – White bread

just bungs your bowels up! Nettle tea and prunes will get everything moving. (**4**) a – Quinoa is a complete source of protein. (**5**) d – I recommend you eat aduki beans several times a week to lose weight. They seem to have a natural diuretic effect by getting rid of excess body fluids. (**6**) b – Blackcurrants contain about 3 times more vitamin C per 100g than oranges. (**7**) a – Hemp seeds contain a 1:1 ratio of the essential omega-3 and omega-6 fats. Olive oil contains some omega-6 fats, while avocados contain some omega-3 fats. Both olive oil and avocados are good sources of monounsaturated fats, which have been shown to be beneficial to heart health. (**8**) c – Tahini (sesame seed paste) contains 380mg of magnesium and 680mg of calcium per 100g. (**9**) b – Oats are a good source of slow-releasing carbohydrates that keep blood sugar and energy levels stable for longer than fast-releasing carbohydrates, such as those found in white flour products and processed breakfast cereals. (**10**) c – Grapefruit has been shown to increase enzymes involved in both phases of liver detoxification.

Superfood of the day

Sprouts

I don't mean Brussels sprouts, although Brussels are good for you too. I am talking about the sprouting process of soaking, germinating the seed and finally eating the growing live sprouts. The end result is a star superfood and digestion-helper like no other. Sprouts are a simple snack and an easy addition to soups, salads and stews. You can find them in health food stores and supermarkets, or grow your own. My favourites are sunflower seed sprouts. Chickpeas are a cinch to sprout too, and make for an amazing chewy snack. Just soak them in water for 24–48 hours and hey presto, they will start to sprout.

Day 7 end-of-day checkpoint

Have you ...

☐ Promised yourself you'll think 'Carrot' all the way?
  (Instead of Stick!)

☐ Identified the Demotivators or Sabotagers in your life?

☐ Prepared a list of responses for when the Sabotagers
  try to steer you off your path?

☐ Taken Gillian's Quick Quiz?

Keep it up – you're looking good. Until tomorrow ...

DAY 8 AFFIRMATION TIME

Welcome to Day 8 and the start of your second week on Boot Camp. You have a lot of tools to work with now, so please make sure you continue with:

>> Log Book
>> Goals
>> Time Management
>> Positive thoughts
>> Exercise

Today we add a new tool: Affirmations.

AFFIRMATIONS (POSITIVE ONES ONLY!)

I want you to make contact with your inner self. Years ago, I used to hear people say that they 'needed to find themselves'. I never knew anyone was lost. I really didn't know what they meant. With time, age, wisdom and practice, you start to totally get it. As a mum myself now, for example, I have found that the demands of work, kids, husband, the home, paying the mortgage and just living life often mean I run the risk of very little time for myself and for recognition of me. I'm sure you understand what I am talking about here. Everyone at some point feels the same way. You need to schedule out the time to actually do something each day just for you.

The first step is to take note of the conversations you have with yourself. The fact is that we converse with ourselves more than with anyone else, and we do it all the time, every day, throughout the day. You may not even realize all your inner talk, but it goes on constantly. And it can be very negative.

For example:

'Oh, I should have gone to the gym today.'
'I'm too fat.' Or 'I'm too thin.'
'My hair is a mess.'
'I feel unsuccessful.'
'I'm so tired.'

This list could go on for ever. And then there is the added element of other people's criticisms and negative comments about you. When left unchecked, this takes its toll.

Make no mistake about it: your body and mind respond to what you tell them, and feel the energy from which you approach them. If your messages come from a perspective of anger or negativity versus compassion and loving kindness, these are the very vibrations that are absorbed into your biochemistry and your subconscious. You need to take very seriously any messages that you give yourself, whether silently or aloud. Therefore, it is imperative that your inner talk is kind and loving in vibration and positive in words in order to serve you well.

'LET GO' EXERCISE

Starting today, I want you to change your inner talk to ensure that the energy is kind to you and the words are positive. So first feel love for yourself, always. You can certainly notice any negative feelings and thoughts, but then say to yourself, *'Now let it go'*.

You can do this every day in order to recondition yourself to allow you to let go of any negativity. I find the evenings, before going to bed, as good a time as any to do this simple 'let go' exercise. By noticing your stuff and formulating the intention to let go (with kindness), you grow as a person.

Next I want you to rid yourself of the words *'should'* and *'could'* in relation to your personal life and health. These words signify regrets and disharmony and have no intrinsic meaning for a good healthy body and mind. You don't need to do the 'should' or 'could' thing. It does not serve you.

RECONDITION YOUR MIND

Finally, we get to specific positive affirmation training. You will discover here how to retrain your mind and your body responses away from the negative self-talk. The way to override negative self-talk is by repeating positive affirmations. To affirm means to state that something is true, correct and absolute. Many successful people use positive affirmations all the time to help them believe in themselves, whether they do it consciously or subconsciously – but they do it to achieve their success.

My definition of 'success' is to achieve the body you wish, the health you want, the love you desire, the fulfilment you crave, and to be who you really are in your life. By now you'll have realized that Boot Camp is all about positivity, so it'll come as no surprise that the affirmations you're going to make today are going to be positive absolutes.

TASK 1: YOUR AFFIRMATIONS

The strongest, most effective affirmations are those that are personal to you. So I can't write yours for you, although I can give some examples. I want yours to be specific and meaningful to YOU.

Start by looking back at the goals you've written in your **Log Book**. Maybe some of those could form the basis of an affirmation. Or maybe you want something more general about the sort of person you are and your qualities. Think about the areas in your life where you tend to doubt yourself the most – and now re-frame them.

Some examples:

'I am a strong, fit person.'
'I am capable.'
'I am a wonderful person.'

Or simply:
' I love being me.'

Or, even simpler:
'I am love.'

Now it's your turn. Take a fresh sheet in your **Log Book** and come up with two or three positive affirmations that mean something to you. What positive statement feels right for you? You can choose one affirmation or a few; it is your choice.

Now what do you do with these positive statements? Quite simply, you say one of your affirmations to yourself whenever you need to hear it. State it firmly and confidently. Believe it. Feel it. You can say it out loud, then softly, then in a whisper and then in your head. Say it when you're driving, when you're brushing your teeth, when you're exercising, before and after meals, when you're trying to resist temptation, when you're frustrated, when you're elated. Your affirmation(s) can bring you balance.

State your affirmation(s) as you wake in the morning and just before you go to bed. You can write them on sticky notes and place them around your home and workplace as reminders. When you write down your affirmation in black and white with pen on paper, you increase the energy and the power.

A final note: don't feel you have to share your affirmations with anyone if you don't want to. Your affirmations are for you and you alone. If you don't mind your family or your colleagues hearing or reading them, that's fine. But some people like to tease or make disparaging remarks about things they don't understand. So there's nothing wrong with keeping schtum.

NOSTRIL BREATHING

To help you strengthen focus through Boot Camp, please practise the following exercise every single morning. Find somewhere you can sit quietly, undisturbed, for a few minutes. Now …

01 Open your right palm. Use your thumb to close your right nostril. Then breathe in deeply, slowly and fully through your left nostril, for a count of 6.

02 Keeping your thumb in place, use your ring finger to close your left nostril, so both nostrils are now plugged. Hold your breath in for a count of 6.

03 Now lift your right thumb from your right nostril and breathe out through this nostril, again for a count of 6.

04 Once you have fully exhaled on one side of your nostril, start to breathe in again through your right nostril, for a count of 6.

05 Close your right nostril and hold for a count of six, then release your ring finger from your left nostril and breathe out for a count of 6.

06 Breathe in again through your left nostril and start the cycle all over again.

In effect, you are going from right nostril to left nostril.

Always make your breathing quiet, slow and even. Repeat the cycle for a total of about 5 minutes. This technique is so simple once you've done it a few times. This exercise can help to quiet your mind and refocus your intentions. When you focus on the breathing, hold and count, your mind is occupied or preoccupied; so in essence you are being freed from all excess thinking. In effect, you give a rest to your brain as well as an infusion of oxygen to the cells. It is relaxing and regenerating at the same time.

Here's the Short Version for quick reference:

» In through the left (nostril).
» Hold.
» Out through the right.
» In through the right.
» Hold.
» Out through the left.
» In through the left.
» And so on ...

Superfood of the day

Quinoa
Quinoa (pronounced 'keenwa') contains **all** the essential amino acids (the building blocks for protein), is calcium-rich, and cooks in no time at all to give you a delicious soft nutty flavour. Serve quinoa up as a hot cereal, a pudding, a cold grain in salads or add it to soups and stews.

Day 8: end-of-day checkpoint

Have you ...

☐ Used your Boot Camp Tools daily?

☐ Drafted positive personal Affirmations?

☐ Verbally stated your Affirmations when you needed a boost?

☐ Done Nostril Breathing?

These simple tools create a firm base from which to succeed. And I am affirming that I will see you tomorrow, bright and early. You do the same. Tomorrow we get to grips with creating balance in your life.

DAY 9 THE PIE OF LIFE

It's Day 9 – can you believe it? You are doing it!

Doesn't time fly when you're living healthily! And talking of time, you'll remember this from Day 4, when I had you fill out charts detailing where every last minute of your day was going. Boot Camper, you need to take a serious look at how you are coming along with time allocation, because today you re-prioritize your life. And you need to be placed at the top of the priority list.

Since Day 4, your **Time Management** skills must have improved and you are now procrastinating less (or not all) and fitting far more into your day. That's an excellent achievement. But what I want you to work on now is balance and taking control of your destiny.

TASK 1: THE PIE OF LIFE

An uncle used to say to me, *'Everything in moderation – that's the way to feel good.'* He actually had a point.

But my revised motto is: *'Everything in Balance.'*

This is the secret of health on all levels. I want your body, your mind and your spirit to be striving for or in perfect balance. This will serve you well. An astrologer once told me that my quest for balance was related to my astrological birth sign of Libra. But I say it also has to do with my knowledge of physiology and the human condition. When you are in balance and in harmony with yourself and your surroundings, you have the best chance of being healthy. So please let's work on getting your life into balance.

In this pursuit, I would like you to use a Pie Chart to represent the various segments of your life (see page 240 to get you started). The idea is that the chart will flag up areas that may be out of balance. Taking note of this balancing act will help you to recognize the key areas, so that you may get on to the path that feels best for you.

In your **Log Book**, draw your own personalized version of the Pie, divided into as many or as few segments as you like, each referring to different areas of your life. Colour in each of these segments, starting from the middle (zero), according to how much time you spend on this area of your life. For instance, if you work full-time and often put in overtime, too, your work segment will be coloured right out to possibly number 10. And if you can't even remember what a hobby is, let alone when you last spent time on one, that segment will score a big, fat, colourless zero. But remember, your Pie is personal to you. It may have only six segments, or eight. You may class hobbies and 'me time' as the same thing, or count exercise as fun.

Once you have completed the Pie Chart, I'd like you to consider how satisfied you are in each of the areas. Perhaps work takes up a lot of your time, for instance, but that might be OK because you find your career satisfying. Maybe family takes up most of your day, and that could be fine because you feel that you want it that way; but if all the attention on family means you are craving more 'me' time, then you know that the Pie is out of balance in this particular segment.

At the end of the day, it comes down to how you feel in your gut, your tummy, your heart and soul, or, as I say, 'in your huesos'. You need to feel it. You and only you can decide if the various areas of your life are in or out of balance. Over the course of my Boot Camp, please feel free to revisit this Pie whenever you want. You will find that by taking the moment to look at yourself, the segments will start to balance out, so that eventually it becomes a flowing smooth ride.

For now, just be aware of how your time is spent, and what adjustments you could make so that every area is satisfying, or at least most areas.

TASK 2: BOOK YOUR CLEANSE DAY

Grab your diary, flick ahead to roughly 3 weeks' time, and write 'Gillian's Cleanse Day' in big bold letters over one of the days. Yes, you may have guessed it. I'm asking you to do a 24-hour Cleanse. The reason I want you to book it now is to give you advance notice to properly schedule a day for peace and quiet at home. So take a day off work, send the kids to their grandparents, pack your partner off to play golf … whatever, please do it. I will take you through the Cleanse Day at the next level, page 134.

Superfood of the day

Kale
Don't be afraid of the dark green leafy kale. It brings about the same kind of scary reaction as when I suggest people try seaweed. No need, though. This is a wonderful healthy food, fab for weight loss. Kale has a crinkly shape, but when steamed the flavour is succulent. Raw, it tastes good too, and I happily juice kale into my carrot juice to get an extra zap of liver-supporting minerals.

GILLIAN'S INSTANT HEALTH SNACKS

Stay with me and there will never be an excuse to fall off the wagon.

I won't let you! My objective is to ensure that you have all the tools to stay focused, inspired, motivated and on the straight and narrow.

I'll problem-solve every step of the way to make it simple and easy for you. For example, worried about snack-attacks? No problem. I've got solutions for every kind of snack attack.

SNACKS ON THE GO

Kiddies' box of raisins

Banana

Apple

Snack-pack of dried apricots

Small packet of unsalted, unroasted mixed nuts

Goji berries

SAVOURY SNACKS

Handful of mixed, dry-toasted seeds (sesame, sunflower and pumpkin)

Brazil nuts

Sliced pepper and carrot sticks with hummus or guacamole

Mug of miso soup

1 cup of homemade popcorn (no sugar, butter or salt!)

SNACKS FOR A SWEET TOOTH

Homemade berry smoothie

Baked sweet potato

Handful of dates

Handful of figs

3 passion fruits

Mango slices

Fruit salad

Dried fruit

Pomegranate seeds

Day 9 end-of-day checkpoint

Have you …

☐ Reviewed Time Management charts and spotted areas you need to work on?

☐ Coloured in your Pie of Life?

☐ Booked your Cleanse Day?

☐ Made a note to stock up on some healthy snacks?

Remember, the more balance you create in your life, the fitter, healthier and happier you can be, the more energy you'll have and the easier it will be to find harmony and real fulfilment in each day.

DAY 10 SEEING IS BELIEVING

It's Day 10, Boot Camper, and you're now into double digits, a full Ten Days!

You are to be congratulated and commended for your perseverance, determination and good work! Today, you will be flexing your muscles. No, I'm not talking bicep curls (that comes tomorrow!). I mean flexing your Visualization Muscle.

I call it a 'muscle' because I really believe that every cell in your body responds to everything that goes on in your mind. Visualization isn't just a mental exercise. It gets whole-body, whole-life results.

Visualization is where you start with a thought and then allow the image to further be visualized to new levels, almost as if it is all real: see the outcome you desire; watch it play out; feel it in your skin and gut; smell it, hear it, touch it. To strengthen your Visualization Muscle, I want you to virtually experience the outcome with all your senses: sight, taste, smell, hearing, touch. In other words, you BECOME it.

Let's give it a try.

TASK 1: VISUALIZING YOUR GOALS

Take your **Log Book** and refer back to the **Primary** and **Daily Mini-Goals** you set on Day 3. Rewrite your **Primary Goal** here:

....

(remember, it must be in the present tense, as in 'I am fit', for instance).

Now you're ready to start visualizing it. In time, you'll be able to do this anywhere: in the queue at the supermarket, on the bus, in the shower, in bed, literally anywhere, any time; although please not while driving or operating heavy machinery!

To get started, though, make it easier by finding a nice quiet relaxing place: maybe in the bath, in bed, on the sofa, or in your favourite spot in the garden. Close your eyes. Take a few slow, deep breaths in and out to relax. Listen to your breath for a couple of minutes to clear and calm the mind.

Start to visualize your **Primary Goal** as a reality (because it is). I'm going to use the example of fitting into a favourite dress, but you will of course substitute your own **Primary Goal**. You can also use the same technique for **Daily Mini-Goals**.

You imagine yourself going to the wardrobe to take out the dress. Perhaps on the way you catch sight of your fit, healthy, slender body in the mirror and like what you see. Your partner catches sight of you and you hear his appreciative remarks. You take the dress and slip it over your head. It slides on with ease, fitting perfectly. The material feels luxurious against your skin. You smooth it down with your hands. Taking another admiring glance in the mirror, you add some jewellery, perhaps a pair of heels, a spritz of your favourite perfume, breathing in its heady aroma. You look great! And you smile ...

You get the picture? You literally create the whole scenario. Just don't forget to add as many details as you can: what room you're in, what sounds you can hear, what the weather is like, everything. In your new virtual world of visualization, you can create anything you want, exactly and specifically the way you want it. It is your world and you have the power.

The more you strengthen your Visualization Muscle, the more easily you will be able to transfer the energy from visualization to actual physical manifestation.

A couple more examples in brief:

If your goal is running a race or entering a sporting event, see yourself crossing the finishing line, accepting your medal. Visualize yourself in all the right gear, putting in your training and enjoying it. Feel the sweat running down your forehead and arms. Hear yourself breathing as you run. Notice how fit, energetic and content you feel.

If your goal is eating more healthily, see yourself preparing a delicious meal and sitting down to enjoy it. Visualize and actually hear the sound of the knife on the chopping board; smell the delectable aromas coming from the oven; listen to the gasps of delight as you serve the complete ravishing dish to your guests. And, of course, experience how wonderful and satisfying it tastes. Yum!

Don't fret if it seems hard at first, or if your mind keeps wandering. It is the same with all muscle training, whether we're talking here about your biceps muscle or your Visualization Muscle – with practice you will succeed.

So start simple, build up, and most important, do it regularly. Two minutes of vivid visualization is better than no minutes, and eventually 2 minutes becomes 5; it is consistency in this muscle-strengthening that will bring about reality actualization. In other words, your dreams will become real (because they already are when you apply my principles).

You can apply this concept to any and every aspect of your life, including work, money, love, leisure, family and more.

And just for the record, everyone has the ability to strengthen this muscle. Don't let anyone tell you otherwise. We all have this power. You now need to decide to use it, develop it, expand it, and live it.

If you do one thing today, you must try this visualization exercise. I'm not asking you to accept it, or asking whether you want to do it or not. I am very simply telling you to just go and start doing it today and every day. Trust me.

MAKE TIME TO MEDITATE

Regular meditation can help everything from your stress levels to your bowel movements to your blood pressure. Studies have indicated that people who practise meditation (or what I would like to call 'exercises in calming the mind') are less likely to have heart attacks, for example, and more likely to live longer. This is an essential way to keep stress levels low when on a weight-loss programme. When you get excessively stressed, the body may produce chemicals which can lead to hormone imbalances, causing further weight gain. When you meditate, you are simply practising 'relaxed awareness', peaceful focus on your breath and noticing your body in the present moment – not reliving the past or thinking about what's going to happen in future. You can quietly notice your breath and your body at any time, anywhere. That is your meditation treat for bringing physiological balance and for healing the body.

Superfood of the day

Millet

The gluten-free grain millet is a fabulous digestive aid.
Chronic indigestion, gas, bloating, burping, belching, bad
breath all respond well to millet. Cook millet with cauliflower
and then mash the two together: the texture is similar
to potatoes. See page 195 for my Millet mash recipe.

Day 10 end-of-day checkpoint

Have you ...

☐ Practised visualizing to strengthen your Visualization
Muscle?

☐ Added Meditation into your day?

Visualize your body dancing up a
storm, as tomorrow we kick that
bahookee of yours into touch. It's
time to fitten up, Boot Campers.

DAY 11 LET'S GET MOVING

Training Day. There are no two ways about it, exercise
is essential to good health on all levels.

Keeping fit burns calories to maintain a healthy weight.
Regular exercise increases your cardiovascular fitness,
promoting a strong heart and good lung capacity. It
strengthens your bones, builds muscle, increases flexibility.
Physical fitness is linked to a lower risk of obesity, as well
as prevention of heart disease, depression, diabetes,
osteoporosis, arthritis, even cancer. That's just for starters.
In short, physical fitness exercise is your life source. It is an
absolute must – there's no way to get around it. And we can
make it fun!

What's more, exercise releases feel-good hormones called
endorphins which move through your body and boost mood.
So you'll be better, look fitter and feel happier too.

Now, there are two ways to start moving:

01 CHANGING YOUR DAILY ROUTINE

Build more movement into your daily routine. It's easy to do,
and you only need to keep the changes up for about a week
before they become a habit. For example, ditch the car and
walk to work. Or park further away from your destination
and walk the distance. Take the stairs, not the lift; walk
up escalators; hide the remote control so you have to get up
to change TV channels. Keep your body moving *every day
as much as possible.*

02 MAKING TIME FOR SPECIFIC FUN ACTIVITIES

If you associate exercise with drudgery or hard work, today's
the day to put an end to that type of thought. You can decide

today to change any negative cognitive associations with exercise. Start by thinking of exercise as fun. Conjure up a happy image of playtime, like outdoor breaks at school when we were little. The important thing is that you start to think about the possibilities when it comes to exercise and then take action. Most important is that you need to find a form of exercise that works for you. This is your chance to do something for yourself.

Here is a sample list of possibilities:

Aquaerobics
Archery
Badminton
Bowling
Boxing or kick boxing
Canoeing
Circus skills
Climbing
Cricket
Cycling
Dancing (ballet,
    ballroom, ceroc, disco,
    Latin, pole, salsa, tap)
Fencing
Football
Golf
Gym exercise classes
Hiking

Ice skating
Jogging or running
Martial arts
Mountaineering
Netball
Pilates
Running
Skipping
Strength-training exercises
    (such as Body Pump or
    'Legs, Bums & Tums'
    classes)
Swimming
Tennis
Volleyball
Walking
Yoga

This list is by no means exhaustive. Ask around and see what your friends or relatives do that they enjoy. Could you join their club or class and see if you like it? Think about what activities you've enjoyed in the past. This is your chance to connect with the 'child' in you. Feel who you are and what you would like. If you liked team sports at school, why not find your local adult hockey or netball or football team? If you're more of a solitary exerciser, try the gym or maybe a yoga class. Cycling or boxing or dancing the salsa may also fit the bill.

TASK 1: CHANGES AND FUN

For today's task, think about and feel different ways you could include more: (1) Daily Routine Changes, and (2) Fun Activities into your life.

Then take out your **Log Book**. On a fresh sheet, I want you to write down three daily changes you'll commit to doing, and three fun activities you'll try out. For example:

Daily Routine Changes:

01 If a journey would take less than 5 minutes in the car, I walk it.

02 I will no longer use the lift at work. I use the stairs only.

03 Instead of emailing colleagues in my office, I walk to their desks.

Fun Activities:

01 I take that trampolining course (or I buy a trampoline!).

02 I go swimming once a week.

03 I take the whole family for a walk every Sunday to the park and we play with a frisbee!

These become your Exercise Promises.

SOME WORDS OF MOTIVATION

It's my job to make sure you get results. But you must do the work. I can't run the marathon for you! This is Boot Camp, after all, so you need to be fully engaged and proactive with our process. Please continue to imagine and visualize and feel the new you: you look great; you feel young; you are healthy; everyone wants your body. Stay focused.

But for those times when there could be a slight blip – for instance, it might be raining outside, or you're tired, or whatever – here are some motivational tips to get you through:

›› **Get the right kit.** You'd be amazed at the difference a new pair of trainers, some trendy yoga gear or a cool-looking cycling outfit could make. If you look the part, you feel the part, and then you are truly embodying all of it.

›› **Find an exercise buddy** – a friend or relative who wants to shape up, too. Agree to exercise together for one or two of your weekly sessions. You'll be less likely to break the commitment if it means letting someone else down. And it's also a whole lot more fun with a buddy.

›› **Sign up to a sports club** or join a team. Many people find they push themselves harder, enjoy exercise more and are more likely to turn up if there's a social element to their chosen form of fitness. And that doesn't include going to the pub afterwards!

>> **Bulk-buy a course of lessons**. Pay in advance for a series. You'll probably save money, plus you won't want to miss a class, as you'll already have paid for it.

>> **Start doing exercise as a family.** Whether it's coaching football for your kids and their friends, cycling through the park, rounders, whatever, wouldn't you rather be a fit parent who joins in than one who watches from the sidelines?

>> **Set goals.** Sign up for that sponsored walk or enter a competition. You could even set yourself mini-goals, such as not getting out of breath when you climb the stairs, or swimming 10 lengths of the pool without stopping.

THE WIDE-AWAKE SHAKE!

Here's a quick fun exercise to do every morning – guaranteed to shake out the cobwebs and get your energy flowing. As silly as you might feel, find yourself a space where you can shake your wrists, your arms, one leg then the other, shake your torso, jiggle your shoulders. It's a bit like the 'hokey-kokey' that you might have played at parties as a kid; great exercise and a lot of fun, too. If you find yourself laughing, so much the better. Jump up and down a little, all the time taking a deep breath and exhaling sharply. Don't do it to the point of dizziness – pace yourself, never overdo it. Do it for a few minutes. When you stop, you may sense a 'fizziness' in your body. That's your energy waking up – your 'chi' is flowing. Just remember: 'Shake till you're fizzy, but not dizzy!' Let yourself go!

➤➤ **Reward yourself.** Remember the list of mini-rewards you drew up on Day 3? When you stick to your daily exercise plan, or meet a goal, you may have a reward.

Superfood of the day

Hemp, raw shelled hemp seeds

Raw shelled hemp seeds are protein-packed and deliciously tasty with a nutty flavour, easy to eat and digest and so versatile. Aim for at least 2 tablespoons of raw shelled hemp seeds 3 or 4 times a week. Toss them into salads, soups, smoothies, stews, casseroles, dips, or eat them by themselves as a fab snack. Check out hemp flour for making breads and pancakes; and you can even find hemp pastas in health food stores – delicious and amazing!

Day 11: end-of-day checkpoint

Have you ...

☐ Written down all the Daily Changes you could add into your life routine?

☐ Written down all the Fun Activities that interest you?

☐ Committed to 3 of each that you'll definitely try?

☐ Thought about Motivational Tips when you have a blip?

☐ Tried my Wide-Awake Shake?

Remember, please keep your body moving!

DAY 12 CONSCIOUS EATING

Welcome to Day 12! You are doing it! And doing so well.

Since you signed up for my Boot Camp, your experience of eating has been gradually shifting. Food is life, and the quality of *your* life will depend on the food you eat, as well as *how* you eat it. And the tools you are learning here can be applied to so many other aspects of your life: family, relationships, career, work. At Boot Camp, we use the physical energy of food as the starting point to springboard to all other levels of your life. In other words, we start with the food as an easy and simple common denominator and then the sky is the limit.

The *old* line, *'You may have had a complex relationship with food'*, is a thing of the past. Maybe you craved nasties you knew were bad for you, then felt guilty and ill after eating them; or maybe you didn't really think about what you were eating, just grabbed whatever was handy while you got on with work or kids or chores, and so you just ignored yourself. It's like you were sweeping yourself under the carpet.

The new you now looks at yourself with love, enjoying the whole eating experience, every minute of it, starting today. From now onward, the eating process is a positive and conscious one. I want you to notice each morsel of food and slowly feel every sensation in your mouth. Be conscious and aware and thankful for each titbit of food as it moves through your mouth and then your throat and into your stomach. And don't take a mung bean's notice of anyone who moans on at you that you are taking too long to eat. Just carry on regardless.

You may wonder, *'What does consciousness have to do with my weight loss?'*

Consciousness means to be self-aware and aware of your environment. First, when you are self-aware you make better choices with food, and everything else in your life for that matter. Second, self-awareness brings more calm and peace to the body. You become more balanced on both physiological and psychological levels. When the mind and body are calm, for example, your digestion works better, food is metabolized at a more efficient rate, the bowels flow more smoothly.

Cravings, over-eating and binges can all be avoided if you learn to shop for, prepare and eat your food consciously, with a positive attitude. When a person eats in response to cravings they are not fully conscious, but reacting to whatever stimuli happen to come their way. They are at the mercy of every influence. The aim of consciousness sets you on the path to healthy weight loss.

TASK 1: SHOPPING MINDFULLY

You can learn to develop your 'sensory awareness' when shopping in order to advance your consciousness. At some point over the next couple of days, go out to the food store and buy some food. Just before you enter the shop, take a few deep breaths in and out, and just listen to your breath. You don't need to think about anything. I want you to just listen to your breath and feel the sensations of your body: feel the air currents around your skin; notice your skin; notice your feet against the ground; hear the breath entering your tummy, breathing slowly; imagine the breath is *peacefully* filling your entire body, and then just stay focused on the area around your tummy button.

Just before you walk into the food shop, quietly say to yourself:

'I allow myself to feel the energy of the food.'

You are now ready to walk into the shop (Don't worry if you get some funny stares! You could always do our little thing *behind* the shop!).

Do not analyse or think about what's good or bad. No judgements; less or no thinking for this task please. The point here is to calm the mind and move along the shop aisles from the perspective of your body's 'feeling centre', your **intuitive energy.** We want to be feeling, rather than thinking, during this task. You may have certain practicalities in mind, such as the need to create a meal to satisfy yourself and your family. But that's as far as the practical side goes. I want the rest to be determined by your intuition. Walk along the produce aisle where the fruits and vegetables are presented. From your body's feeling centre, notice which fruits and veggies attract you and vice versa. You can then start to make food choices according to how you feel.

When you get home, make a note in your **Log Book** about how this task felt, what foods you selected and whether they were unusual choices. The more you practise this exercise each time you go to the food shop, the more you develop your intuitive sensory awareness for food.

TASK 2: CONSCIOUS MEALTIMES

From now on, I also want you to be mindful of every meal or snack you make, from the first stage of preparation to the final bite. As soon as you enter your kitchen, be mindful of what you're doing. This second task is to be done with your next meal:

01 Select your ingredients consciously, with full awareness of yourself and of the food. Notice and appreciate how the food looks, feels and smells. Feel the energy of the food.

02 Prepare your food with care, attention, love and gratitude. Perhaps your family or guests would like to join in and share the experience with you. Make it fun. Or if you're alone, enjoy being in the present moment, making it no less special because it's for you.

03 Give your food the respect it deserves for the nourishment it's about to give you. Arrange it beautifully on a plate. Set the table. Even if it's just a solo snack. Treat a mealtime as a sacred moment.

04 Be conscious of every mouthful. Appreciate and notice the look, aroma, texture, taste, even the crunch or slurp you might make.

05 Feel gratitude that you are able to enjoy this life-giving, delicious food.

GET SPROUTING

Sprouts are the tiny young green plants germinated from seeds, nuts, grains, beans and pulses. Add them raw to salads, throw them into stir-fries right at the end of cooking, even just snack on a handful. Sprouting is a low-cost easy way to infuse plenty of nutrients into your body. If you have little kids, they'll love the fun of growing sprouts.

Once you've mastered alfalfa sprouts (see below), experiment with others, such as mung beans, chickpeas and soya beans.

You will need:

» A pack of alfalfa seeds (from a health food store)
» A large jam jar
» A piece of muslin or cheesecloth about 20cm square
» A large rubber band
» A sieve

How to do it:

» Rinse a tablespoon of seeds well and put them into the jam jar.

» Cover with 2–3cm of boiled, cooled water.

» Cover the jar with your muslin or cheesecloth and secure with the rubber band.

» Leave overnight in a warm, dark place.

» Next morning, tip the seeds out into a sieve. Rinse well. Return them to the jar (without water), re-cover and return to the dark. Repeat twice a day until the seeds begin to sprout.

» Once they're sprouting, place the jar on a bright windowsill for a few hours to give them an energy boost; but then store the jar out of direct sunlight. Tilt it to about 45 degrees so the sprouts grow up the sides.

» When the sprouts are 3–6cm long, they're ready to harvest and eat.

Or you can just buy sprouting trays or even a sprouting machine, which are available nowadays, and that's a whole lot easier than all these steps. You simply chuck the seeds on to trays, water them and watch them grow.

Superfood of the day

Daikon radish

Daikon is a strange-looking food, but don't let that put you off. It looks like a very long white carrot and I want you to use it in soups and stews. Great for ridding the body of excess mucus. Find it in health food stores and oriental markets.

Day 12: end-of-day checkpoint

Have you ...

☐ Completed Mindful Shopping?

☐ Practised conscious food preparation and eating?

☐ Vowed to develop your sensory awareness with food?

☐ Tried sprouting seeds?

Happy eating! See you tomorrow.

DAY 13 GOING OUT GUIDE

You've made it to Day 13! We have nearly completed the intensive 14 days of my Boot Camp. And you are still going strong to tell the story!

Let's explore solutions to some of the difficulties you could encounter over the coming weeks and months, and how to overcome them with confidence and gusto when you go out.

In my private practice, clients have worried unnecessarily about various potential issues that might arise. For example, socializing and mixing with 'normal' people once they get on to the Gillian McKeith path could be a challenge: they're not sure if it's OK for them to eat a meal at a restaurant, or meet friends at a pub, or order a takeaway. Or they might get muddled up and unsure about exactly what foods to choose when going out on the town.

SOLUTIONS

01 Of course you can have a social life!

What do you think I am, some sort of diet dictator? (Well, don't answer that!) But even I occasionally might receive an invitation to a dinner, a party, a drink at the bar – could you believe – Go figure!

You will be amazed at my response, because I am here to tell you that you can accept that invitation with pride and gratitude: yes, go along and enjoy yourself. You heard right. Go ahead and accept that occasional invite. As a Boot Camper who is just about to graduate, the rules for you can be slightly loosened. You now have the tools to have a fantastic night out, without over-indulging or feeling bad about it afterwards.

02 **A friend keeps pressuring you to go out, but you don't actually want to. What do you do?**

As a Boot Camper, you now know that you are in control of your own life. Check in with your body, your gut, your sensory feeling centre. How do you feel? Do you want to go out or stay in? It's your call, it's your life. You must ascertain how you really feel at your core, not what you are thinking in your head, but what you are feeling really, and then that is your decision made easily.

It's called *'keeping it real'*. If friends try to persuade you otherwise, just be flattered – they want your company. But stick to your guns; state your desires firmly and clearly, always with kindness. Remember Day 7? Be who you really are.

03 **Not sure what you can and can't eat when going out?**

Here's the deal. You can eat what you want. You choose. All I ask is that you make your choices mindfully, in accordance with conscious eating. Recognize that it's a special occasion; give yourself permission to choose what you like. Enjoy the evening and get back on track the next morning.

QUICK TIPS

▶▶ Don't starve yourself before going out. Treat it as a normal meal. Deny yourself all day in anticipation, and you'll dive straight into the bread bowl, gorge on four courses and end up feeling bloated, gassy and down on yourself.

▶▶ Mineral water, juice, even herbal teas are all beverages you can drink instead of alcohol or fizzy sodas at your local.

▶▶ Drink a glass of still water (no ice) as soon as you arrive at your going-out place. It'll make you feel fuller and provide hydration in what are often stuffy venues.

» When your guests order, do not feel that you need to match them course for course. Order what you feel like. Get just a main course if that's all you fancy. You need not order a starter and a dessert and who knows what else, just because you think it's the thing to do. You're not obliged to share their bottle of wine if you'd rather not. You could always be the one to order your meal first, if it means you're not swayed by the choices of others. Boot Camp is about empowering you to stand on your own two feet and be who you really are, so you can now be truly comfortable in your own skin.

» If the main courses don't suit you, do what I do: just order a combination of starters and side dishes, and voilà! you create your own main course. Be creative.

» Don't be shy when going out. You are the customer, so feel free to ask questions and offer instruction to the restaurant servers. They are in the business of serving you. If you want your fish grilled and not fried, for instance, or soup to be cream-free, or even the bread-basket to be taken away to avoid temptation, simply open your mouth and speak the words. (*Just hope you don't get banned from the eatery like I was once!* But in life, to be who you really are, you need to take a chance – and stand your ground.)

» Eat mindfully, even at the pub lunch. Admire your meal when it arrives, savour every mouthful, feel every texture against the palate, give thanks. Chew very calmly, eat quietly; and put down your cutlery as much as possible between mouthfuls and in between courses to really help slow down your eating. Don't worry if your culinary companions are racing through their dishes – their digestion will suffer and they, not you, will be the ones farting like troopers.

92 going out guide

But you can be assured that you are the Boot Camper who is now the real Commander of your own life.

>> Irrespective of what your mother may have told you when you were little, you need not eat everything on your plate. Mum may always have been right about most things, but not this one. Sorry, Mum. Eat the amount of food that feels right for you.

>> Don't be afraid to order dessert when going out, especially if the restaurant is known for fab puddings and if you really, really want it. But please take some time for the main part of your meal to digest before tucking in to the sweets. The portions of desserts at most restaurants are often far too big, rich and sweet. You probably really just want a taste, so I suggest you share with one or two others in your party. It really does the trick. You get the best of all worlds when you share your pudding with another. Alternatively, ask the restaurant if they could do you a 'half portion'.

TASK: PLAN AHEAD

Take a look at your diary to determine if you are going out any time soon; you can even check if there is a lunch meeting at work. But a personal rendezvous would be ideal. I want you to plan ahead and think about how you can adapt and apply all the principles we've just discussed. Remember, practice makes perfect. So if you have nothing planned, your task is to get something in the diary soon; find someone to go out with.

Then I want you to implement some of the Quick Tips above.

If you plan it out in advance as I suggest here, I know you are learning and developing the art of being proactive in your life – taking control. I don't want you to just react to any stimuli and surrounding influence that happens to come your way like a mindless amoeba; instead I want you to take the reins. This is why you now need to be conscious and proactive in your life. And you will not only lose the weight, guaranteed, and look and feel great too, but you will fly to new heights in all aspects of your future. This is my promise to you.

Superfood of the day

Fennel

Traditionally fennel has been used as a slimming food. Chewing the seeds is reputed to reduce hunger pangs and the desire for sweet foods. Fennel is thought to help the liver and pancreas with the digestion of fats and sugars and to help the mobilization of stored fat into the bloodstream. Fennel also has diuretic properties, meaning it can help reduce excess water in the body.

Day 13: end-of-day checkpoint

Have you ...

☐ Checked out the Solutions for Going Out?

☐ Learned your Quick Tips?

☐ Found a friend to Plan Ahead?

☐ Reviewed the Best and Worst of Going Out?

Bon appétit!

THE BEST AND WORST

ITALIAN

The Worst! Creamy sauces, thick pizza bases, cheesy toppings, bread sticks.

The Best! Minestrone soup, olives, salads, tomato-based sauces, grilled white meat or fish dishes – dressing on the side.

INDIAN

The Worst! Anything battered, fried, naan bread, creamy sauces, piles of white rice.

The Best! Mild vegetable curry, spicy salads, lassis (special smoothies).

CHINESE

The Worst! Deep-fried anything, added sugar or MSG.

The Best! Vegetable dishes, chicken, noodles, tofu stuff.

BRITISH

The Worst! Rich sauce, salty gravy, deep-frying or battering, huge bread baskets or potato portions.

The Best! Seasonal, local, organic veggies, grilled or steamed fish and white meat, salads, non-creamy soups.

AWARD FOR THE BEST

My personal favourite is … JAPANESE, one of the healthiest foods around. Miso soup, sashimi, salads, vegetable, seaweed and tofu dishes and buckwheat or brown rice noodle soups are good choices. My only words of caution: white rice isn't very nutritious so don't *just* go for sushi rolls. Go easy on the soy sauce, as it's high in sodium.

DAY 14 GRADUATION DAY

Wow, you've done it!

This has been a great time, one which kick-starts your whole new future. I may be your Boot Camp Sergeant-Major, but you are now clearly the Commander of your own life! I now loosen my grip, because I'm confident you've got what it takes to go it alone as a Boot Camp graduate.

To keep on track, you must continue to write in your **Log Book**: note your food intake; manage exercise time; always recognize how you are feeling. You know the score by now. It's important to keep up the daily notes and records, to stay mindful of how you're living your life.

The key here is to become aware of yourself, your feelings, taking note of who you really are, facing yourself full on, accepting and loving yourself just the way you are, and allowing openness and transformation. This is the road to freedom, peace, contentment, ultimate health and a really great body too!

TASK 1: TAKE STOCK AND REFLECT

You may recall that back on Day 1 I asked you to answer a series of questions to assess your **General Health Profile** and I asked you to **Log Your Progress**. I now want you to return to these questions (see page 15) and answer them again, so that you may realize the change you've undergone.

» How do your responses differ, if at all?

» What do the differences tell you about how far you've come in the past couple of weeks?

 96 graduation day

» What areas do you still need to work on?

This is a good exercise to do whenever you need to check your progress – please complete the **Profile** again at any time in the future.

TASK 2: REASSESS YOUR INTENTION

Look back to your **Declaration of Intent**.

01 Have you stayed true to your **Declaration of Intent** or are you moving towards it?

02 Has your intention changed since you started Boot Camp? Maybe you feel you've already surpassed it, or perhaps your focus has changed?

If your answer to number 1 is yes, even if you still feel you're a long way off, simply recommit to this statement. If your answer to number 2 is yes, work out your new **Declaration of Intent** or refine it. Write it down and make this the focus of the next 4 weeks.

TASK 3: RE-EVALUATE YOUR GOALS

Now turn your attention towards your **Goals** – the ones you set on Day 3.

01 How are you doing with your Goals – Primary and Minis?

02 Have you come up with some inspiring rewards for meeting your Goals?

03 How many Goals remain outstanding and do they still seem important to you?

04 As you've changed your habits and become healthier, have any new Goals occurred to you?

TASK 4: LOOK WITHIN YOU

Take a moment to think and feel where you are:

» What have you most enjoyed over the past 14 days?
» What is most surprising?
» Which foods have you enjoyed?
» And not enjoyed? (Let them go.)
» Any new discoveries about yourself?
» What changes have you noticed, physical, mental or emotional? What have you been particularly good at?
» What have you learned for life?

TASK 5: WRITING ASSIGNMENT: POSITIVE REALIZATIONS

Make a list of all the positive experiences you've had over the past 14 days. Keep this list safe. Refer to it whenever you need a reminder or a motivational boost.

Superfood of the day

Dandelion greens

Fabulous mineral-rich liver supporter with diuretic properties; a great source of B vitamins too. Dandelion tea and even dandelion coffee are available in health food stores.

10 MOTIVATIONAL TIPS

Feel free to rewrite or cut out my Motivationals and place them anywhere it might help you: on the fridge door, in your bedroom, on a bathroom mirror, at your work desk.

01 Gillian's energy is with me.

02 Don't think so much, just be in your body.

03 Don't ask so many questions. Just do it!

04 Did you drink water today?

05 You won't shrink that backside by sitting on it!

06 Peckish? Bored? Fed up? Then do some fun fitness stuff.

07 Repeat after me: *'I love fruits and vegetables.'*

08 Repeat after me: *'I love all of me.'*

09 Take control of your body and your health.

10 You Can Do It.

Day 14: End-of-day checkpoint

Did you ...

☐ Re-do your General Health Profile and Log Progress?

☐ Reassess your Declaration of Intent?

☐ Re-evaluate your Goals?

☐ Take note and look within yourself?

☐ Write down Positive Realizations?

☐ Use the Motivationals?

☐ Know that you can re-do the intensive part of Boot Camp as often as you want?

Be proud of yourself, I certainly am. Congratulations! Wishing you Love and Light.

Gillian xx

GILLIAN'S BOOTCAMP
CERTIFICATE OF
GRADUATION

This is to certify that

_____

has graduated from Gillian McKeith's
Intensive Boot Camp and is now healthier
than ever and well on the road to success!

Congratulations!

Gillian M Keith

GILLIAN MCKEITH

BOOT CAMP
LEVEL TWO

THE NEXT LEVEL

THE HEALTH FACTOR TESTS

Now you are a Boot Camp Graduate you can take some time over the next few weeks to focus on any specific health factors that might need extra help. Work through the following quick questionnaires to identify your priority health factors (the 3 with the highest scores) and start to incorporate the suggestions into your diet and lifestyle.

Health factor: adrenal stress

01 Do you often feel tired when you wake up, with that dragged-through-a-hedge feeling even after you have had 7–8 hours' sleep? 10

02 Do you feel drowsy during the day and experience a mid-afternoon energy slump? 5

03 Are you an anxious or nervous person? 5

04 Do you have a lot of weight around your middle whereby you look like you drink beer or are wearing a doughnut? 20

05 Do you suffer from frequent colds and infections? 5

06 Do you have high or low blood pressure? 20

07 Do you suffer from chronic fatigue, weakness, lethargy or lack of motivation, difficulty sleeping? 10

08 Do you have cuts or serrations in the middle of the tongue or a reddish tip? 10

09 Do you crave salt? 5

10 Do you use caffeine, alcohol or nicotine regularly to keep yourself going? 10

>> **Score**

ADRENAL STRESS ACTION PLAN

When adrenal function is out of balance, more stress hormones are released. This excess hormone release can cause blood sugar imbalances that may lead to further weight gain. Lack of sleep, and a diet high in sugary foods and low in B vitamins compromises adrenal function.

>> **Avoid stimulants, including caffeine, alcohol and nicotine.**

>> **Avoid foods that upset blood sugar,** including added sugar, refined carbohydrates and packaged foods containing added sugar.

>> **Avoid using too much salt.** Use herbs, spices, miso and tamari soy sauce instead.

>> **Eat lots of green vegetables.** These contain magnesium, which gets used up in times of stress.

>> **Eat whole grains** for their B vitamin content, needed for energy and adrenal health.

» **Eat berries, kiwis and grapefruit** for their vitamin C content. Stress depletes the adrenals of vitamin C.

» **Herbs to support the adrenals include** rhodiola, ginseng, astragalus and ashwagandha.

» **Eat asparagus with the tips and dip into hummus.**

» **Herbs to aid relaxation include** chamomile, lemon balm, lime flowers and skullcap.

» **Take regular, moderate exercise daily.** Avoid exercising in the evening, as this can trigger stress hormones that interfere with sleep.

» **Go to bed before 11 p.m.** Sufficient rest and relaxation are important for adrenal health.

» **Learn to meditate.** During meditation both the mind and body are completely relaxed.

» **Check out the blood sugar section too (see opposite).**

Recipes:
Roasted butternut squash soup (page 159)
Red fruit blitz (page 147)
Quinoa porridge (page 145)
Aduki bean bake (page 163)
Savoury vegetable rice (page 198)

Health factor: blood sugar balance/energy

01 Do you struggle to get up and get going in the morning? 5

02 Do you get shaky, dizzy or irritable if you don't eat often enough? 10

03 Do you suffer from excessive thirst? 10

04 Do you suffer from energy dips during the day? 5

05 Do you frequently wake up in the night or in the early hours of the morning? 10

06 Do you have frequent cups of tea, coffee, soft drinks and sugary snacks to keep you going? 10

07 Do you need to urinate frequently? 10

08 Do you crave sugar or carbohydrates? 10

09 Do you tend to put on weight around the middle (as opposed to hips and thighs)? 20

10 Do you get exhausted when you exercise or sometimes find you simply cannot exercise for love nor money? 10

>> **Score**

BLOOD SUGAR ACTION PLAN

Blood sugar levels impact energy and weight. Every time blood sugar levels are raised, insulin is released to take the sugar from the blood to the cells. Insulin is a storage hormone that likes to store sugars as fat. The more insulin released, the more fat you are likely to lay down. Stable blood sugar levels give you steady energy and can help keep weight regulated too. It's worth getting a check-up from your GP, as higher scores could suggest a possible pre-diabetic condition, developing diabetes and/or the metabolic syndrome (insulin resistance). Insulin imbalances are not helpful to weight balance.

➤➤ **Avoid sugar, refined carbohydrates, alcohol, fizzy drinks, white pastas, sweeties and caffeine.**

➤➤ **Eat 6 meals a day.** That means breakfast, snack, lunch, snack, dinner, snack.

➤➤ **Eat complex carbohydrates**. Complex carbohydrates break down and release their sugars slowly, giving a steady trickle of energy. Brown rice, quinoa, oats, millet, buckwheat, lentils and beans are all good sources.

➤➤ **Combine protein with carbohydrates**. Protein slows down the release of sugars from carbohydrates, thus keeping blood sugar more stable.

➤➤ **Include cinnamon, fenugreek, turmeric, onion and garlic in your cooking.**

➤➤ **Get moving.** Exercise improves the cellular response to insulin.

➤➤ **Chromium, B vitamins, magnesium, zinc, vitamin D and manganese** are all needed for blood sugar stability.

» **Useful herbal supplements include ginseng, bitter melon, glucomannan and gymnema sylvestra.**

Recipes:
Quinoa and mixed bean salad (page 187)
Lentil salad (page 182)
Mock-a-leekie soup (page 158), followed by
   Avocado stuffed with black-eyed peas (page 205)
Chicken and vegetable curry (page 168)
Fatoush (page 180) with brown rice

Health factor: detoxification

01 Do you suffer from frequent headaches? 5

02 Do you get skin problems such as greasy skin, acne, itchy bottom, skin rashes or eczema? 10

03 Do you have trouble digesting fatty foods? Burping, farting and body smells would be a clue? 15

04 Do you have light-coloured, yellowish or sticky, mucusy poos and/or a yellow or mucky white coating on your tongue, or a swollen tongue? 15

05 Do you suffer from IBS, constipation, diarrhoea, gallstones, PMT? 10

06 Do you have any allergies or food sensitivities, throat mucus or a runny nose? 10

07 Do you often have a bitter or metallic or yucky taste in your mouth (especially in the mornings)? $\boxed{10}$

08 Do you frequently drink alcohol, fizzy drinks, colas or coffee, or do you smoke or take drugs? $\boxed{10}$

09 Is your diet high in sugar, refined carbohydrates and processed foods? $\boxed{10}$

10 Do you often go to bed later than 11 p.m.? $\boxed{5}$

>> **Score**

DETOXIFICATION ACTION PLAN

The liver is the major organ of detoxification, but other body parts that play a detox role are the kidneys, lymph, skin, lungs and bowel. The body stores toxins in various body parts, including fat cells. Supporting your body's natural detox can help the breaking down of fat. Do as much as you can to lighten the toxic load for your liver and gall bladder.

>> **Avoid alcohol, caffeine, nicotine, artificial additives, soft drinks and sweeteners.**

>> **Start the day with warm water with a squeeze of lemon.**

>> **Avoid fatty and fried foods.**

>> **Have grapefruit for breakfast.** Grapefruit can speed up detoxification. Check with your GP if you are on medication.

>> **Drink water, veggie juices or herbal teas every day.**

Dandelion coffee and nettle tea are particularly beneficial to the liver.

》 **Have a salad every day.** Raw foods are cleansing and nourishing.

》 **Do regular 1 or 2 day cleanses** (see page 134).

》 **Get to bed by 10.30 p.m.** The liver and gall bladder are most active between 11 p.m. and 3 a.m.

》 **Take the herbs milk thistle and coptis.** They come in tincture form or capsules, so could be added to teas or smoothies.

》 **Dry skin brush before you shower.** This gets the lymph and waste products moving.

Recipes:
Fruit salad (page 143)
Cleanser in the raw (page 150)
Crunchy walnut coleslaw (page 178)
Cleanser juice (page 146)
Cabbage and fennel with lemon and thyme (page 191)

Health factor: digestion

01 Do you frequently suffer from bloating or flatulence? 10

02 Do you have difficult or irregular bowel movements, with either diarrhoea, constipation or IBS type symptoms? (A good indicator of healthy bowel movement is twice a day.) 10

03 Do you suffer from indigestion or heartburn? ☐10

04 Does your tongue have a yellow, white or dirty-coloured coating? Or a line down the middle, teeth marks round the edges or cuts/serrations? ☐10

05 Do you often suffer from bad breath? ☐5

06 Do you feel as though food sits in your stomach for a long time after you have eaten? ☐10

07 Are your stools exhibiting any of the following: smelly, greasy, leave skid marks on the loo, slimy, thin and shreddy in appearance, pellet or pebble shaped, like rabbit droppings? ☐15

08 Do you generally eat white refined carbohydrates rather than whole grains? ☐10

09 Is your diet low in fruit and vegetables (i.e. fewer than 5 portions a day)? ☐10

10 Have you taken any courses of antibiotics recently? ☐10

>> **Score**

DIGESTION ACTION PLAN

The digestive system breaks down foods, assimilates nutrients and eliminates waste products. If there is a back-up in your digestive plumbing, that's not good news. Nutrient absorption needed for metabolism and energy is compromised. This can cause all sorts of health problems, including weight gain and lack of energy.

>> **Eat whole grains.** These contain fibre, needed for a healthy digestive tract. Examples include oats, millet, quinoa, brown rice, buckwheat and rye.

>> **Eat fruit on an empty stomach.** This avoids fermentation and gas.

>> **Follow food-combining rules.** Eat animal protein with vegetables or salads. Eat beans and pulses with grains and vegetables.

>> **Avoid irritants.** These include chillies, pepper, alcohol, caffeine and additives. Some people find citrus fruits a problem.

>> **Avoid foods to which you are intolerant.** Wheat and dairy are common culprits.

>> **Use herbs and mild spices.** Ginger, coriander, cumin, cinnamon, caraway, chervil, peppermint, fennel and dill can all aid digestion.

>> **Take slippery elm bark powder mixed in juice or water 3 times weekly.**

>> **Chew thoroughly until your food is liquid before you swallow it.**

>> **Relax when you eat.** Avoid rushing around straight after eating.

>> **Take digestive enzymes with meals.**

>> **Supplement with probiotics such as acidophilus.**

RECIPES:
Mango mad smoothie (page 147)
Millet mash and onion gravy (page 195)
Watercress soup (page 161)
Grilled sea bass with herb sauce (page 171)
Sprouting salad (page 200)

Health factor: female hormones

Questions for women

01 Do you suffer from PMS symptoms such as breast tenderness, water retention, cravings, irritability, mood swings? ☐10

02 Do you suffer from menopausal symptoms such as hot flushes, vaginal dryness, irritability, mood swings, excessive sweating, night sweats? ☐10

03 Are your periods irregular, excessive or prolonged? ☐10

04 Do you suffer from acne that relates to your menstrual cycle? ☐10

05 Do you lack sex drive or interest in sex or have you had difficulty getting pregnant? ☐10

06 Do you suffer from depression, fatigue or anxiety? ☐5

07 Have you been diagnosed with any conditions related to female hormonal imbalances, such as endometriosis, fibroids, fibrocystic breast disease or polycystic ovarian syndrome? 15

08 Do you have thinning hair on your head and/or facial hair? 10

09 Do you have osteoporosis? 10

10 Do you carry excess weight around the hips and thighs? 10

>> **Score**

FEMALE HORMONES ACTION PLAN

The hormone levels of oestrogen and progesterone fluctuate over the course of a menstrual cycle. Menopausal symptoms are caused by a reduction in female hormones. The female hormones, especially oestrogen, tend to encourage fat deposition, especially round the hips and thighs. In turn excess fat on the body can lead to imbalances in the female hormones.

If you have queries about your hormonal status, ask your GP to run some hormone tests.

>> **Avoid sugar, alcohol, caffeine, excess salt and refined carbohydrates.** They have a disruptive influence on the female hormonal system.

>> **Include phyto-oestrogens in your diet.** These are plant oestrogens that can help to balance oestrogen levels. They are found in soya, linseeds, alfalfa, pulses and whole grains.

>> **Avoid xeno-oestrogens.** These are poisonous oestrogens that can upset hormonal balance. They are found in plastics, pesticides and unfiltered water.

>> **Drink oestrogenic herbs as teas.** Fenugreek, liquorice, red clover, fennel and sage are all useful.

>> **Eat green vegetables.** These are good sources of magnesium and vitamin B6, both of which are needed for female hormone balance.

>> **Eat shelled hemp seeds, flax seeds, pumpkin seeds and sunflower seeds.** These all contain the essential fats needed for a healthy hormonal system.

>> **Support your liver and bowel.** Together these are responsible for the removal of old hormones. See sections on detoxification and digestion (pages 109 and 111).

>> **Move that bahookee and do regular exercise.**

>> **Herbs that can help with female hormone balance include** agnus castus, dong quai, motherwort, black cohosh and false unicorn root. It is best to check with a practitioner as to which is best for you.

>> **Supplements of magnesium, vitamin B6, vitamin E, Evening Primrose Oil and fish oils** can all be helpful.

Recipes:
Spinach and tofu with mixed leaves and watercress dressing
   (page 199)
Edamame and pea soup or Sage soup (pages 155 and 152)
Marinated tofu with lemon sauce (page 172)
Cooling salad (page 192)
Moroccan chickpea salad (page 183)

Health factor: male hormones

Questions for men

01 Do you suffer from low sex drive or loss of interest in sex? [10]

02 Do you suffer from impotence or erectile dysfunction? [15]

03 Do you have problems with urination or increased urination? [10]

04 Do you suffer from lack of energy or drive? [5]

05 Do you lack muscle tone or have your muscles diminished? [10]

06 Do you have a tendency to put on fat rather than muscle? [10]

07 Do you drink more than 21 units of alcohol a week and/or smoke? [10]

08 Do you often feel irritable or angry? [5]

09 Do you often feel depressed and unmotivated? [5]

10 Have you got a low sperm count or poor sperm quality? [20]

>> Score

MALE HORMONES ACTION PLAN

The main male sex hormone is testosterone. As men age, their levels of female hormones such as oestrogen tend to rise, while testosterone levels decline. Imbalanced sex hormones in men can lead to an excess of oestrogen, which results in men losing muscle and gaining fat and can even lead to the development of the increasingly common man boobs.

Get your GP to run a hormone test if you are unsure about hormonal status and its effects.

>> **Eat 2–3 tablespoons of pumpkin seeds daily** – these are a great source of zinc, which is needed for male sexual health. Other good sources include flax seeds, whole grains, pulses, fish, eggs and lean meats.

>> **Avoid sugar, caffeine, alcohol and refined foods** – these can upset insulin levels, which in turn can interfere with male hormone balance.

>> **Eat nuts and seeds daily.** Hemp, flax, sunflower, pumpkin and sesame seeds and their oils are all good sources of the essential fats and vitamin E needed for hormone balance and healthy sperm production.

>> **Eat 3 Brazil nuts a day for their selenium content.** Selenium is vital for healthy sperm production.

>> **Eat organic.** Many pesticides can upset sex hormone balance.

>> **Eat whole grains daily** – these are rich in fibre, which is needed to remove old hormones from the body. Brown rice, millet, quinoa and oats are all good sources.

>> **Take regular exercise** – exercise is generally beneficial to hormone balance.

>> **The herb saw palmetto** can help balance testosterone levels.

>> **Nutrients to support the male reproductive system** include zinc, selenium, vitamin E and L-arginine.

>> **Check Adrenal Stress Action Plan** (page 105).

Recipes:
Scrumptious stuffed peppers (page 176)
Herb omelette (page 144)
Layered Mexican salad (page 181)
Really easy chicken stir-fry (page 170)
Mediterranean-style cod stew (page 174)

Health factor: food sensitivity

01 Do you suffer from known allergies: to pollen, dust, feathers or a particular food? 15

02 Do you frequently suffer from bloating or flatulence? 15

03 Do you suffer from digestive problems such as constipation or diarrhoea, or have you been diagnosed with IBS? 15

04 Do you feel drowsy after eating certain foods? 10

05 Do you suffer from frequent headaches, migraines,

aching joints or water retention? 10

06 Are there any foods that you crave or wouldn't want to live without? 5

07 Do you ever get a racing pulse after eating or a tongue or mouth ulcer? 10

08 Do you get dark circles under the eyes? 5

09 Do you suffer from itching or other skin problems such as eczema? 10

10 Do you suffer from hyperactivity or depression? 5

>> **Score**

FOOD SENSITIVITY ACTION PLAN

Food sensitivities can lead to a wide range of symptoms. You may crave foods to which you are sensitive when you first take a break from eating them, but this will soon pass, so stick with it.

Food sensitivities can lead to water retention, which can make you heavier and more puffy. They can also lead to cravings and weight gain.

>> **Establish which foods are causing a reaction.** You can either just avoid those foods you suspect are causing problems or you can have a food intolerance test. You can check your own pulse, too, before and after eating a meal. If your pulse count per 60 seconds has increased by 10 beats or more, you may be reacting to that particular food.

>> **The most common problem foods are** wheat, dairy products, yeast, soya, corn, citrus fruits, shellfish, sugar.

>> If you do stop eating any food, **make sure you eat a varied and balanced diet**. Eating too much of one food can lead to an intolerance.

>> **Replace the foods you are avoiding with equivalents.** Wheat and the other gluten grains can be replaced with quinoa, millet, buckwheat, brown rice, wild rice and red rice. Cow's milk can be replaced with rice or oat milk.

>> **Strengthen your immune system.** A weakened immune system can often cause you to react to foods. When your immunity is strengthened, you become less reactive. See **Immunity Action Plan,** page 129.

>> **Eat a varied diet.** This is the best way to avoid becoming intolerant to more foods. Ideally rotate foods on a 4-day basis. If you suspect that you are reacting to a food but are baffled as to where to start, **get a food sensitivity test done**.

>> **Herbs to aid digestion include** ginger, cardamom, peppermint, fennel, dill and caraway.

>> **Avoid gut irritants such as** alcohol, caffeine and some painkillers and medications.

>> **Support digestion and absorption with digestive enzymes.**

>> **Take 5gm of L-glutamine on an empty stomach daily to heal the gut.**

» **Slippery elm powder mixed in juice or water before meals is helpful too.**

It is a good idea to get tested for food sensitivities. For more information go to *www.gillianmckeithclinic.com*.

Health factor: heart and circulation

01 Do you frequently drink alcohol, caffeinated drinks and/or smoke? `10`

02 Do sugar and refined carbohydrates feature regularly in your diet? `10`

03 Do you add salt to your food or often eat packaged, processed or fast foods? `10`

04 Is your diet high in saturated or processed fats from dairy products, processed foods and fatty meats? `10`

05 Do you have a sedentary lifestyle, taking little or no exercise? `10`

06 Do you suffer from shortness of breath upon any exertion? `10`

07 Do you often suffer from stress or anxiety? `10`

08 Have you been diagnosed with any cardiovascular imbalances such as high blood pressure, high cholesterol, high triglycerides, high homocysteine or atherosclerosis? `20`

09 Do you have circulatory problems such as cold hands and feet, leg cramps, easy bruising or varicose veins? [10]

10 Are you overweight or do you carry excess weight around your midriff? [20]

HEART AND CIRCULATION ACTION PLAN

The cardiovascular system comprises the heart, veins, arteries and capillaries. Being overweight puts you at huge risk of cardiovascular problems.

>> **Avoid** fatty meats, dairy products, sugar, salt, refined foods, fried foods, margarine, processed and packaged foods, cigarettes, caffeine and excess alcohol.

>> **Eat 8 portions of fruit and vegetables a day.** These contain nutrients and antioxidants that can protect the cardiovascular system.

>> **Eat pumpkin seeds, shelled hemp seeds and flax seeds,** for their omega 3 content. Other sources include oily fish, walnuts and avocados.

>> **Eat olives and olive oil** – these contain mono-unsaturated fats that have been shown to have a beneficial effect on cholesterol ratios.

>> **Eat oats** – rich in soluble fibre, needed to remove excess cholesterol and waste from the body. Other good sources of fibre include brown rice, quinoa, millet and buckwheat.

»» **Eat a largely vegetarian diet.** Vegetarian sources of protein include pulses, nuts, seeds, quinoa and amaranth.

»» **Replace salt with herbs and mild spices.**

»» **Drink nettle tea** – it has a slight diuretic effect that can reduce blood pressure.

»» **Take up yoga, meditation, tai chi or breathing exercises to lower stress levels.**

»» **Exercise.** Anything that raises the heart rate to an extent where you are breathing deeply but still able to have a conversation is ideal.

»» **Maintain a healthy weight.**

»» **Useful herbs include hawthorn and gingko biloba.**

»» **Useful supplements include fish oils and magnesium.**

If you suspect you may be at risk of any cardiovascular problems, get checked out by your GP.

Recipes:
Easy oats (page 143)
Olive tapenade (page 208)
Baked salmon parcels (page 164)
Celeriac and carrot purée (page 192)
Green beans with warm cherry tomatoes
    and garlic (page 194)

Health factor: hypo-thyroid

01 Do you tend to feel the cold more than most? 10

02 Do you suffer from constipation? 10

03 Do you tend to have dry skin? 5

04 Have you experienced thinning hair on your head or loss of hair from your outer eyebrows? 15

05 Do you have a slow pulse rate, under 60 beats per minute? 10

06 Do you feel tired on waking, even after 7 or 8 hours' sleep? 10

07 Do you tend to put on weight easily and find it hard to lose weight? 15

08 Do you generally feel lethargic? 10

09 Do you feel mentally sluggish? 5

10 Do you have a poor appetite? 10

>> **Score**

Under-functioning Thyroid Action Plan
Hypothyroidism refers to an under-active thyroid, meaning the thyroid does not produce sufficient quantities of thyroid hormones. The thyroid hormones play a big part in

controlling our metabolic rate (the rate at which we burn up calories for energy) and body temperature. A deficiency can result in fatigue, weakness, constipation, depression and weight gain, because the thyroid controls the metabolic rate. An under-functioning thyroid means a slowed metabolism and a reduced rate of calorie burning.

If you suspect that your thyroid could be slightly under-active, get your GP to run a thyroid test. Often test results come back within normal levels even when the thyroid is not functioning optimally. This is because the parameters of what is considered normal are very wide and the tests do not necessarily include all the relevant markers of health. If your test results are normal but you have lots of the symptoms above, follow the dietary and lifestyle advice in the recommendations section.

If you have an underactive thyroid, check with your GP before embarking on any nutritional programme.

>> **Eat sea vegetables regularly but in small quantities.** Include nori, kelp, dulse, kombu and arame.

>> **Eat 2–3 Brazil nuts a day.** Brazil nuts contain selenium, which is needed for thyroid hormone production.

>> **Use flax seed oil in salad dressings.** The oil in flax seeds is particularly beneficial for the endocrine system, including the thyroid.

>> **Avoid wheat.** The gliadin in wheat can be toxic to the thyroid, so is best avoided. Some people do best without the other gluten grains as well (oats, rye, barley, kamut and spelt).

>> **Avoid RAW cruciferous vegetables, soya and millet.** These can all suppress thyroid function. The cruciferous vegetables are fine if cooked, and fermented soya in moderation is also fine (natto, miso, tempeh and tamari).

>> **Avoid sugar, refined carbohydrates, processed foods, alcohol, salt, caffeine and dairy products.**

>> **Avoid fluorine and chlorine.** Fluorine is found in many toothpastes, tap water and tea. Chlorine is found in tap water and swimming pools. Filter your water and use fluoride-free toothpaste.

>> **Drink 8 glasses of pure water daily.**

>> **Support the adrenals.** See the section on the adrenals (page 104).

>> **Take 500mg of L-tyrosine 20 minutes before breakfast and lunch.**

>> Take moderate exercise daily.

>> **Support your adrenals,** as thyroid problems often follow on from adrenal depletion.

Recipes:
Nori sushi rolls (page 185)
Spiced rice pudding (page 212)
Skinny soup (page 160)
Aduki beans with red onion and corn salsa (page 177)
White bean mash (page 204)

Health factor: immune system

01 Do you suffer from frequent colds and infections? 10

02 Do you take a long time to recover from infections? 10

03 Do you have white spots on your nails or have hangnails? 5

04 Do you ever suffer from swollen lymph glands (under the arms, in the groin or below the ears)? 10

05 Do you suffer from allergies and sensitivities, hives, elevated yeast levels or Candida albicans, or have you ever had glandular fever? 10

06 Do you often get boils or styes? 10

07 Do you suffer from inflammation in any part of the body? 10

08 Do you eat fewer than 5 pieces of fruit and vegetables a day? 10

09 Do you eat sugar and refined carbohydrates regularly? 10

10 Do you often take antibiotics, or have you taken many in the past? 10

>> Score

IMMUNITY ACTION PLAN

Your immune system is responsible for protecting you from disease and infection. Antioxidants from food are an important part of the immune system's armoury. When the immune system is struggling, food sensitivities are more likely. These can lead to water retention and cravings for more of the offending foods, both of which contribute to increased weight.

>> **Eat at least 8 portions of fruit and vegetables a day.** Eat as wide a range of colours as you can, to maximize the range of antioxidants you take in.

>> **Get juicing.** A glass of vegetable juice daily will provide your immune system with a whole host of antioxidants.

>> **Avoid sugar** – it suppresses immune function.

>> **Avoid alcohol and caffeine** – both can deplete you of nutrients.

>> **Eat pumpkin seeds.** These are rich in zinc, which is needed for healing and repair.

>> **Eat 2–3 Brazil nuts a day.** These are rich in selenium, which is needed for immune function.

>> **Replace saturated fats with essential fats.** The essential fats have an anti-inflammatory effect. They are found in oily fish, walnuts, hemp seeds, pumpkin seeds, flax seeds and the cold pressed oils of these seeds.

>> **Avoid dairy products.** These are mucus-forming. Avoid

anything else to which you may be intolerant. See section on food sensitivities (page 119).

>> **Take a green superfood daily.** Wheat grass, barley grass, spirulina and blue green algae are all rich sources of the nutrients and antioxidants needed for immune function.

>> **Sprouted broccoli seeds** have been found helpful.

>> **Drink water, herbal teas and veggie juices regularly.**

>> **Astragalus, pau darco, echinacea, Siberian ginseng, lemon peel and ginger are supportive herbs.**

>> **Take regular exercise.** Overdoing exercise can suppress the immune system and put you at risk of injury, but moderate exercise improves immune function.

>> **Supplement with 1,000mg of vitamin C twice a day and 15mg of zinc daily.**

RECIPES:
Baked shiitake mushrooms (page 142)
Moroccan chickpea salad (page 183)
Mung stew (page 175)
Berrytastic smoothie (page 147)
Crunchy courgette and carrot salad (page 193)

Health factor: mind/mood

01 Do you often feel low or depressed for no apparent reason? 10

02 Do you lack a sense of purpose in life? `10`

03 Do you suffer from anxiety or panic attacks? `10`

04 Do you have trouble sleeping? `10`

05 Do you often feel lethargic or unmotivated? `10`

06 Do your moods swing up and down? `10`

07 Is there a family history of depression or mental health problems, or have you ever been diagnosed with a mental health problem? `15`

08 Do you have any cuts or markings or spots on the tongue? `5`

09 Do you over- or undereat when stressed or worried? `10`

10 Do you use alcohol, caffeine, nicotine or other drugs to make yourself feel better? `10`

›› Score

MIND/MOOD ACTION PLAN

Diet and lifestyle play a big role in how you feel and the stability of your moods. Consult your GP and ask about counselling if you suffer from regular or severe depression or mental instability. Depression and mood swings can lead to comfort eating, irregular appetite and weight gain.

Make sure you are keeping your daily food/mood/exercise diary and see if any insight to your moods is revealed.

» **Keep blood sugar levels stable.** Blood sugar stability can have a major impact on your mood. See the section on blood sugar (page 107) for more information.

» **Avoid caffeine, alcohol, nicotine, additives, artificial sweeteners and street drugs.**

» **Avoid wheat and dairy**, which can both affect brain function and mood.

» **Eat oily fish 2–3 times a week.** These contain omega-3 fatty acids, which have been shown to improve many aspects of mental health. Other sources include flax seeds, hemp seeds, pumpkin seeds and walnuts.

» **Eat mangoes. They contain properties that are natural mood elevators.**

» **Eat green vegetables, beans and lentils.** These are high in folic acid, which has been found to be low in those with depressive disorders.

» **Eat Brazil nuts for their selenium content,** which helps to improve mood.

» **Avoid lead, aluminium, cadmium and mercury.** Sources include pollution, amalgam fillings, deodorants, cigarette smoke, some paint, lead water pipes, aluminium cooking utensils and some fish, such as tuna, swordfish and shark.

» **Eat a high-fibre diet.** Fibre, particularly pectin, can remove harmful metals and toxins from the body. Good sources include sea vegetables, apples, plums, Concorde grapes, the pith of citrus fruits, redcurrants and cranberries.

» **Drink 8 large glasses of water and herbal teas daily.** Water is vital for a healthy brain.

» **Exercise daily, preferably in daylight.** Both exercise and daylight can improve mood and energy.

» **Deal with stress.** Yoga, tai chi, meditation, counselling or support groups can all be helpful.

» **Supplement with chlorella**. This can remove metals such as mercury from the body.

» **Supplement with fish oils and zinc.**

RECIPES:
Mixed leaves with brazil nut pesto (page 196)
Beany root vegetable stew (page 165)
Avocado vinaigrette (page 206)
Cacao cream smoothie (page 148)
Buckwheat noodle salad with pok choi and sesame
    dressing (page 184)

CLEANSE DAY

My **Boot Camp Cleanse** is to give you a bit of a clear-out.
It's not a punishment, so banish such thoughts from your
mind now!

Your body is detoxing itself each and every day through
sweat, wee and daily bowel movements. But, and it's a big
fat but, modern life is so polluted that we can all use a bit
of the extra cleanse support. That's where Boot Camp
Cleanse comes in.

24-hour Cleanse

Spend the day at home, uninterrupted by chores or
appointments. Forget trying to cleanse at work, unless you
have a fairy godmother who is willing to show up at your
office at designated times with veggie juices and raw salads.

Be Prepared
Plan ahead. Tell friends and family you're not to be disturbed.
Make a list of everything you will need for Boot Camp
Cleanse day.

The Week Before
Get all supplies *before* Cleanse Day, not *on* Cleanse Day. Be
in bed by 10 p.m. every night the week before your cleanse.

Deeper cleanse option
Make an appointment for a colonic irrigation. It's a bit
like an enema but about 40 times more powerful. To find a
therapist near you, go to *www. gillianmckeith.info/colonic*.
I am not forcing you to get a colonic, but it can help when
there is a history of constipation, headaches, yeast infections,
indigestion, burps, farts, bloating and smelly poos.

THE CLEANSE KIT

EQUIPMENT

Blender

Juicer

Essential oils of
frankincense and lavender

Hot water bottle

Long skin brush with
a handle

Candle

Tongue scraper

DRINKS

Sage tea

Dandelion tea

Nettle tea

Pink grapefruit juice

Milk thistle tincture

Cleavers tincture

FOODS

1 pack of linseeds

1 lemon

125g each of strawberries,
raspberries and cherries

1 pack of celery sticks

4 cucumbers

6–8 large carrots

1 beetroot

1 small piece of fresh ginger

2 avocados

8 spring onions

1 garlic bulb

vegetable bouillon (stock) powder

1 apple

1 fennel bulb

1 lettuce

1 small packet of parsley

1 romaine lettuce

1 bag of rocket

lamb's lettuce

sugar snap peas

chicory

alfalfa and mung bean sprouts

olive oil

hemp seed oil

apple cider vinegar

nori (seaweed) flakes

chervil

THE NIGHT BEFORE YOU CLEANSE
Soak overnight 1 tablespoon of linseeds/flax seeds (same thing) in a large mug of warm water.

THE CLEANSE DAY
» **Before** you leave your bedroom, sit comfortably at the end of your bed or on a chair or on the floor. Breathe in through your nose and out again through your nose. With each breath, gradually start to increase the length of time that you inhale and exhale. If you feel any strain, just return to normal breathing. Breathing out fully is just as important as breathing in fully. Do this for 10–15 minutes.

» Start your cleanse day with a large glass of warm water with a squeeze of lemon juice. Follow this with a mug of nettle tea. This helps to kick-start the liver and bowel.

» Strain the linseeds that were soaking overnight and drink the broth only.

» Follow this with **Red fruit blitz** (page 147).

» Go for a gentle walk somewhere green.

» Mid-morning, make a large vegetable juice. Juice 2 sticks of celery, 4 carrots, 1 cucumber, ½ a beetroot and a tiny piece of fresh ginger. Add 5 drops of milk thistle tincture.

» Before lunch, go for another gentle walk somewhere green.

» When you get back from your walk, drink a large mug of dandelion tea.

>> **Cleanser in the raw** – or **Skinny soup**, if you fancy something warm (see pages 150, 160).

>> Mid-afternoon, make another vegetable juice with celery, fennel, lettuce, parsley and a green apple. Green foods contain magnesium, needed for cellular cleansing. Add 5 drops of milk thistle.

>> Go for a walk somewhere green.

>> Half an hour before dinner, drink a large mug of sage tea.

>> For dinner, have a small cup of your cleanse soup (page 150) and make a green leafy salad using romaine lettuce, rocket, lamb's lettuce, sugar snap peas, chicory, alfalfa and mung bean sprouts. Sprinkle with olive oil, a squeeze of lemon and nori flakes.

>> Mid-evening, it's time for your Fat Flush. Mix 200ml of pink grapefruit juice with 2 tablespoons of olive oil. Add 10 drops of milk thistle tincture and 10 drops of cleavers tincture. Sip this mixture slowly. It's not going to taste great. Then lie down on your left side and gently massage below the right ribs for 5 minutes in a clockwise direction. Switch sides and rest in that position for another 5 minutes. Slowly get up. Please continue to use the milk thistle and cleavers tinctures, 15 drops each in warm water, every day for the next 5 days.

>> Dry skin brushing – start with the feet and brush up the body using firm strokes, always brushing towards the heart. Brush down from the neck and the top of the chest and back. This moves lymph fluid, improving cleansing. It's also a great antidote to cellulite.

>> Run a warm bath, add some mineral salts and 4 drops each of lavender oil and frankincense oil. Soak in the bath for 20 minutes.

>> Light a candle. Position it a foot away from you in a safe place. Sit comfortably either on the floor or on a chair. Close your eyes for a couple of minutes and become aware of every part of your body. Take note of your feet, legs, arms, stomach, then open your eyes and look at the flame of the candle. Breathe in and out through the nose and be aware of the breath. Thoughts may come into your head, but just let them go. Be more of an observer of the thought than IN the thought. Let the thought go, and move your attention back to the flame and the breath. Ten minutes should do it, and now you should get yourself to bed. Position a hot water bottle at the kidney area as you start to relax. Well done for today.

THE DAY AFTER YOU CLEANSE

>> Next morning, start with a glass of warm water and dandelion tea. Follow this with some fruit.

>> For lunch, finish off your cleanse soup from yesterday and follow with a large mixed salad. Combine grated carrot and beetroot with sprouted lentils or any other sprouts and finely sliced fennel. Sprinkle on some chopped parsley and chervil. Mix well with a dressing of hemp seed oil, olive oil and lemon juice. Chew thoroughly and relax while you enjoy the flavours.

WHAT TO EXPECT

After 3 hours – If you feel hungry, drink herbal tea or have a couple of vegetable crudités.

After 6 hours – a headache might kick in if it's going to, but don't expect it, as it may not happen. Reduce headache potential by taking a green superfood such as spirulina or blue green algae.

After 12 hours – Cleansing uses body resources, so if you are feel tired, it's normal. Take it easy and have an early night.

After 24 hours – You are likely to feel energized and clear-headed. Your tongue may be coated; if so, clean it with a tongue scraper and rinse your mouth out well.

THE BENEFITS

Clothes may feel looser and you feel lighter. Cravings are likely to reduce. Sense of taste and smell will heighten. Need for salt, sugar and strong flavours will reduce.

BOOT CAMP
RECIPES

BREAKFASTS

Baked shiitake mushrooms

SERVES 2
PREP TIME 4–5 MINS
COOKING TIME 20–30 MINS
125g shiitake mushrooms
½ teaspoon hemp oil
1 teaspoon wheat-free tamari soy sauce
I large beef tomato, sliced
a pinch of sea salt
1 tablespoon chopped fresh parsley

1. Preheat the oven to 180°/gas mark 4.

2. Remove the stalks from the mushrooms and place them on a baking tray.

3. Divide the oil and tamari between the centres of the mushrooms, then arrange the tomato slices on the mushroom cups.

4. Transfer to the preheated oven and bake for 20–30 minutes.

5. Transfer to 2 warm serving plates and sprinkle with a little salt and parsley,

Easy oats

SERVES 1
PREP TIME 1–2 MINS
COOKING TIME 15–20 MINS

1. Combine 250g of porridge oats with 125ml of water
or rice milk in a pan.
2. Bring to the boil, then lower the heat and simmer for
15–20 minutes. Season with cinnamon and vanilla essence.

Fruit salad

SERVES 1
PREP TIME 5 MINS
1 mango, peeled and chopped
1 banana, peeled and chopped
a handful of blueberries
6 strawberries, chopped
a handful of pomegranate seeds

1. Combine all the fruit together in a bowl and eat.

Herb omelette

SERVES 2
VERY EASY
PREP AND COOKING TIME 5 MINS
4 free-range organic eggs
2 tablespoons cold water
2 tablespoons fresh parsley or coriander
1 tablespoon olive oil

1. Whisk the eggs and water together in a small bowl, then add the herbs and whisk again.
2. Heat the oil in a non-stick omelette pan and pour in the egg. Leave for 30 seconds for the base to set, then, using a spatula or wooden spoon, draw the egg from the outside of the pan into the centre. Repeat all the way round the pan until the omelette looks ruffled and fluffy.
3. Leave the omelette for 30 seconds to set, then loosen the edges and transfer to a serving plate. Divide the omelette in half, and serve with some rocket leaves and/or grilled tomatoes and shiitake mushrooms.

Quinoa porridge

SERVES 1
PREP AND COOKING TIME 20–25 MINS
150g quinoa grains
½ cinnamon stick
235ml water
75ml apple juice

1. Bring 235ml of water to the boil and the quinoa, cinnamon and apple juice. Bring back to the boil, then reduce the heat and leave to simmer for 10 minutes.
2. Turn off the heat and allow the quinoa to stand for 10 minutes before serving.

JUICES

Carrot craze

PREP TIME 5 MINS
6 carrots
2 celery sticks
1 cucumber

1. Push the vegetables through the juicer and drink slowly.

Booster

PREP TIME 5 MINS
3 celery sticks
3 carrots
1 fennel bulb
½ beetroot

1. Push the vegetables through the juicer and drink slowly.

Cleanser

PREP TIME 5 MINS
5 kale leaves
2 celery stalks
a small bunch of lettuce leaves
juice of ½ lemon
1 apple
a small piece of fresh ginger

1. Push all the ingredients through the juicer and drink slowly. (Add the piece of fresh ginger for more of a kick!)

Note for juicing virgins: add an apple to help you adjust to drinking the veggie juices.

SMOOTHIES

Mango mad

PREP TIME 5 MINS
1 mango, peeled and chopped
1 banana, peeled
1 peach, peeled and chopped

1. Blend together until smooth. Serve over a handful of berries or pomegranate seeds.

Berrytastic

PREP TIME 5 MINS
½ punnet strawberries
½ punnet raspberries
1 banana

1. Blend until smooth and creamy.

Red fruit blitz

PREP TIME 5 MINS
125g strawberries, hulled
125g raspberries
125g cherries, stoned

1. Blitz in a food processor or smoothie maker, adding 50ml water if required. Pour over fresh blueberries and blackberries.

Note To slow down the release of smoothies into the bloodstream and give sustained energy, add an avocado or a superfood powder to each blend.

Strawberry delight

PREP TIME 5 MINS
12 strawberries, hulled
2 nectarines
1 pear

1. Add 120ml water to the fruit in the blender and then blend until smooth.

Cacao cream

PREP TIME 5 MINS
120ml rice milk
2 heaped tablespoons cacao powder
1 banana
1 teaspoon cacao nibs (optional)

1. Blend until smooth and drink. Delicious over raspberries.

Note To slow down the release of smoothies into the bloodstream and give sustained energy, add an avocado or a superfood powder to each blend.

SOUPS

10-minute fish soup

Miso is a tremendous source of good bacteria for your intestinal garden. You can never plant enough good, healthy bacteria in your insides.

SERVES 2
PREP TIME 6 MINS
COOKING TIME 4 MINS

1 garlic clove, sliced
1 teaspoon finely chopped or grated fresh ginger
100g white fish fillet, cut into chunky pieces
8 mangetout, trimmed and sliced
½ red pepper, deseeded and sliced
1 pok choi, washed and sliced
2 spring onions, trimmed and sliced
1 sachet of instant miso soup
a handful of beansprouts
a handful of fresh peas

1. Bring 500ml of water to the boil in a large saucepan.

2. Add the garlic and ginger and cook for 1 minute.

3. Add the fish, mangetout and red pepper, bring back to the boil, skim any foam from the surface and cook for 2 minutes.

4. Add the pok choi and spring onions and cook for 1 minute more.

5. Remove from the heat and stir in the miso, beansprouts and peas. Spoon into a large bowl to serve.

Cleanser in the raw

SERVES 4–6
PREP TIME 5 MINS

2 small ripe avocados
2 cucumbers, trimmed, peeled and roughly chopped
   into 3cm slices
6 spring onions, trimmed and roughly chopped
100ml cider vinegar
2 tablespoons olive oil
1 large garlic clove, roughly chopped
6 ice cubes
100ml cold water
1 tablespoon organic vegetable bouillon (stock powder)

For the garnish (optional)

2 spring onions, trimmed and sliced diagonally
1 tablespoon flax seeds

1. Halve the avocados and scoop out the flesh. Place this and the other ingredients in a food processor and blend until as smooth as possible. Serve immediately, sprinkled with spring onions and flax seeds, drizzled with a little olive oil if liked.
2. If not serving immediately, transfer to a bowl and cover the surface with cling film. Eat within 24 hours.

Beef tomato and okra soup

SERVES 2
PREP TIME 5 MINS
COOKING TIME 25–30 MINS
1 onion, chopped
1 leek, finely sliced
2 sticks celery, sliced
1 carrot, peeled and sliced
2 tablespoons olive oil
1 tablespoon water
500ml vegetable stock, or water and a stock cube
6 beef tomatoes, chopped
150g frozen okra, defrosted and sliced
2 spring onions, chopped

1. Place the onion, leek, celery and carrot in a pan with the oil and water, and cook over a low heat for 2–3 minutes to soften the vegetables.

2. Add the stock and the tomatoes, bring to the boil, cover the pan and simmer for 20 minutes. Remove from the heat and allow to cool slightly, then blend in a food processor or blender.

3. Return to the pan, then add the okra and cook for 3–4 minutes.

4. Pour into 2 bowls, scatter with the spring onions and serve immediately.

Sage soup

There's a decent amount of soup here, and that's because I want you to freeze some of it so you have it on hand when you need it.

SERVES 4–6
PREP TIME 5 MINS
COOKING TIME 30–35 MINS

2 red onions, chopped
3 garlic cloves
4 carrots, peeled and chopped
1 head of broccoli, florets only
1 white cabbage, shredded
6 new potatoes
1 litre boiling water
3 teaspoons miso powder
a large handful of fresh sage
a large handful of fresh parsley, plus extra to garnish

1. Place all the ingredients except the sage and parsley in a large pan. Bring to the boil, then cover and simmer for 20–30 minutes. Toss the parsley and sage in at the very end – do not cook the herbs.

2. Remove from the heat and blend until smooth.

3. Spoon into large warm bowls and serve sprinkled with the extra parsley.

Carrot and coriander soup

MAKES 4 SERVINGS (SO YOU CAN FREEZE THE EXTRA)
PREP TIME 8 MINS
COOKING TIME 25 MINS
1 tablespoon extra virgin olive oil
2 medium onions, peeled and chopped
500g carrots, peeled and cut into roughly 5mm slices
1 teaspoon ground coriander
1 teaspoon organic vegetable bouillon (stock) powder
1.25 litres just-boiled water
½ supermarket pack (5g) fresh coriander, finely chopped

1. Heat the oil in a large saucepan and gently fry the onions and carrots for 5 minutes, stirring regularly. Do not allow them to colour.

2. Stir in the ground coriander and cook for a few seconds, then add the stock powder and water. Bring to the boil and cook for 15–18 minutes, or until the carrots are very soft.

3. Remove from the heat and allow to cool for a few minutes before blending with a stick blender or in a liquidizer until smooth. Return the soup to the pan, add most of the fresh coriander and warm through for a couple of minutes until hot, adding more water if necessary to achieve the right consistency. Serve garnished with the rest of the fresh coriander.

Corn chowder with pepper salsa

SERVES 2
PREP TIME 5 MINS
COOKING TIME 15 MINS
1 x 326g tinned sweetcorn
1 x 300g tin of cannellini beans
2 spring onions, sliced
2 sticks celery, sliced
a handful of chives, chopped
a few sprigs of parsley
1 tablespoon white miso paste
400ml vegetable stock or water
Pepper Salsa (see below)

1. Set aside two thirds of the sweetcorn. Place all the rest of the ingredients in a pan and bring to the boil, then reduce the heat and simmer for 5 minutes.

2. Transfer to a blender or food processor and blend until smooth. Pour back into the pan, add half the remaining corn, and add a little more stock or water if required to achieve a thick soup consistency.

3. Make the pepper salsa, using the rest of the corn.

4. Spoon the hot soup into 2 bowls and spoon the pepper salsa into the centre of the soup. Serve immediately.

For the pepper salsa

⅓ tin of sweetcorn
½ red pepper, finely chopped
1 stick celery, finely sliced
2 spring onions, sliced
1 tablespoon cider vinegar
fresh chives, chopped

1. Mix all the above ingredients together.

Edamame and pea soup

The secret of meals in minutes is having a tidy and organized kitchen, with everything to hand. Soya beans are now available frozen in large supermarkets. You can get them in health food stores too.

SERVES 2
PREP AND COOKING TIME 12 MINS
2 sachets miso soup powder or stock cubes
4 spring onions
2 sticks celery
125g frozen soya beans
125g frozen peas
a handful of fresh mint leaves

1. Place the miso soup in a medium-sized saucepan and measure 500ml of boiling water into the pan. Place over a high heat and bring back to the boil.
2. Meanwhile finely slice the spring onions and celery, reserving the green tops of the onions and a handful of celery to garnish. Add the onion and celery to the boiling stock.
3. Add the beans and peas to the pan and return the mixture to the boil. Add the mint, then cover the pan with a lid and leave to simmer for 4 minutes.
4. Remove from the heat and blend until smooth.
5. Spoon into 2 bowls, sprinkle with the reserved spring onion tops and celery and serve.

Note If you are using a glass blender, allow the mixture to cool slightly before blending as it will be very hot.

Fresh tomato and basil soup

SERVES 2
PREP TIME 5 MINS
COOKING TIME 15 MINS
300g fresh tomatoes
1 medium onion, chopped
2 garlic cloves, chopped
1 tablespoon oil
1 tablespoon water
a handful of fresh basil
6 cherry tomatoes, halved, and some basil leaves, to garnish

1. Place the tomatoes, onion and garlic in a pan with the oil and water and cook for a few minutes over a moderate heat to allow the onion to soften. Add 500ml of boiling water, bring back to the boil and simmer for 5 minutes.

2. Remove from the heat, add the basil and blend in a food processor or blender.

3. Pour into 2 bowls and serve immediately, garnished with the cherry tomatoes and basil leaves.

Minted pea soup

SERVES 2
PREP TIME 3 MINS
COOKING TIME 6 MINS

1 large onion, finely chopped
1 teaspoon olive oil
1 tablespoon water
1 teaspoon wheat-free vegetable bouillon (stock)
   powder or stock cube
200g frozen peas
a large handful of fresh mint leaves
nori flakes and a few extra peas, to garnish

1. Place the onion in a medium-sized saucepan with the oil and water cook over a moderate heat for 4 minutes, or until translucent and soft.

2. Add 500ml of boiling water, the peas and the stock powder or cube and simmer for 2 minutes.

3. Add the mint, then remove from the heat and blend until smooth.

4. Pour into 2 soup bowls and serve garnished with nori flakes and a few peas.

Mock-a-leekie soup

SERVES 2
PREP TIME 5 MINS
COOKING TIME 25 MINS
2 leeks, finely sliced
3 carrots, peeled and sliced
2 tablespoons olive oil
500ml vegetable stock
100g oat groats
fresh parsley, chopped

1. Place the leeks, carrots and oil in a pan and add
2 tablespoons of the stock.
2. Simmer gently for 3–4 minutes, then add the rest
of the stock and bring to the boil.
3. Add the oat groats, cover the pan and simmer for 20
minutes. Add the parsley and serve immediately.

Roasted butternut squash soup

SERVES 3–4 (SO YOU CAN SAVE SOME FOR NEXT DAY)
PREP TIME 6–8 MINS
COOKING TIME UNDER AN HOUR

1 large butternut squash
2 medium onions, peeled and cut into thick wedges
2 tablespoons olive oil
2 teaspoons organic vegetable bouillon (stock) powder
2 tablespoons fresh young thyme leaves

1. Preheat the oven to 200°C/gas mark 6. Peel the butternut squash and cut it in half. Discard the seeds and cut the flesh into 3–4cm chunks. Place in a bowl with the onions. Pour over the olive oil and toss well together.

2. Scatter the squash and onions over a baking tray and cook in the centre of the oven for about 40 minutes, until the vegetables are very soft and tinged golden brown. Turn halfway through the cooking time, and do not allow them to over-brown.

3. Remove from the oven and allow to cool for a few minutes before transferring to a food processor. Blend until as smooth as possible, then pass the mixture through a sieve into a clean saucepan.

4. Add 900ml of cold water and the bouillon powder. Bring to a gentle simmer on the hob, stirring regularly, and adding more water if necessary. Stir in the thyme leaves and cook for a few seconds before serving hot in warmed soup bowls.

Skinny soup

SERVES 2
PREP TIME 8 MINS
COOKING TIME 8–10 MINS

2 tablespoons brown rice miso paste
1 heaped teaspoon finely grated fresh ginger
1 garlic clove, peeled and finely chopped
½ fennel bulb, trimmed and diced
75g baby corn, trimmed and thinly sliced
50g mangetout, trimmed and halved lengthways
5 spring onions, trimmed and sliced
1 sheet of nori (toasted seaweed), cut into thick strips

1. Put the miso paste into a saucepan and slowly add 800ml of cold water. Place over a medium heat and stir in the ginger, garlic and fennel. Bring to the boil, then reduce the heat slightly and leave to simmer for 5 minutes.
2. Stir in the baby corn, mangetout, spring onions and nori strips, and simmer for a further 3 minutes, until all the vegetables are just tender. Serve.

Note This soup is delicious served topped with lots of sprouting seeds.

Watercress soup

SERVES 2 AS A STARTER OR LIGHT LUNCH,
FOLLOWED BY A LARGE SALAD
PREP TIME 8–10 MINS
COOKING TIME 18–20 MINS

1 tablespoon cold-pressed sunflower oil or extra
   virgin olive oil
1 medium onion, peeled and finely chopped
2 sticks celery, trimmed and sliced
1 medium sweet potato (around 150g), peeled and cut
   into roughly 2cm cubes
2 garlic cloves, peeled and crushed
2 teaspoons organic vegetable bouillon (stock) powder
1 bag of fresh watercress (100g)
1 tablespoon pumpkin seeds (optional)

1. Heat the oil in a medium saucepan and cook the onion and celery very gently for 3 minutes, until beginning to soften. Stir in the sweet potato and garlic and cook for about a minute.

2. Pour over 500ml of cold water, stir in the bouillon powder and bring to the boil. Reduce the heat slightly and simmer for 15 minutes until the potatoes are soft. Remove from the heat and stir in the watercress. Leave to stand for 2 minutes.

3. Blend until smooth with a hand blender, or allow to cool for 10 minutes then transfer to a liquidizer or food processor to blend.

4. Warm through gently, then ladle into deep bowls and serve sprinkled with pumpkin seeds if liked.

White bean cappuccino

SERVES 2
PREP TIME 10 MINS
COOKING TIME 20 MINS
VERY EASY

1 x 420g tin of organic butter beans
1 onion, finely chopped
1 leek, finely chopped
2 garlic cloves
2 teaspoons organic bouillon (stock) powder
1 bay leaf
2 tablespoons chopped parsley, plus extra leaves to garnish
2 spring onions
a pinch of cinnamon

1. Drain the beans and rinse well.

2. Place the onion, leek and garlic in a saucepan with 4 tablespoons of water and cook over a low heat for 3–4 minutes.

3. Pour in 500ml of boiling water and add the bouillon powder, bay leaf and parsley. Bring to the boil and simmer for 10 minutes.

4. Add the beans and simmer for a further 10 minutes.

5. Remove from the heat, remove and discard the bay leaf and allow to cool.

6. Take out 2 tablespoons of the beans, transfer to a bowl and keep to one side.

7. Blend the remaining soup in a food processor or blender until smooth.

8. Add the reserved whole beans and the spring onions, and serve garnished with parsley leaves and a pinch of cinnamon.

MAIN MEALS

Aduki bean bake

MAKES 2 GENEROUS SERVINGS (ABSOLUTELY DELICIOUS)
PREP TIME 10 MINS
COOKING TIME APPROX.45 MINS

1 tablespoon olive oil, plus extra for brushing
1 medium onion, peeled and chopped
2 garlic cloves, peeled and crushed
1 medium parsnip or squash, peeled and diced
1 large carrot, peeled and diced
1 celery stick, trimmed and sliced
500ml just-boiled water
1 teaspoon organic vegetable bouillon (stock) powder
1 medium leek, trimmed and sliced
165g cooked aduki beans or 1 tin of aduki beans (rinse well)
2 teaspoons cornflour, blended with 1 tablespoon cold water
    to make a smooth paste
1 medium sweet potato, cut into 5mm slices (around 250g
    prepared weight)

1. Heat the oil in a large saucepan and gently fry the onion
and garlic for 3 minutes, stirring occasionally, until soft but
not coloured. Add the parsnip, carrot and celery and cook
with the onion and garlic for 2 minutes, stirring regularly.
2. Pour the water over and stir in the bouillon powder. Bring
to the boil, then reduce the heat and simmer for 10 minutes.
Preheat the oven to 200°C/gas mark 6. Stir the sliced leek
and aduki beans into the vegetable mixture. Return to a
simmer and cook for 5 minutes, stirring occasionally.
3. Add the cornflour mixture and cook for about 1 minute,
stirring, until the sauce thickens. Remove from the heat
and transfer carefully into a 900ml ovenproof dish.
4. Arrange the slices of sweet potato on top of the bean and
vegetable mixture. Brush with a little oil and bake for about
30 minutes, until the potatoes are cooked. Serve with freshly
cooked Savoy cabbage, green beans or broccoli.

Baked salmon parcels

SERVES 2
PREP TIME 10 MINS
COOKING TIME 15–18 MINS

1 medium courgette, trimmed and thinly sliced
1 yellow pepper, deseeded and cut into thin strips
10 cherry tomatoes
2 x 150g fresh salmon fillets (preferably wild or organic)
4 slices of fresh lemon
1 tablespoon olive oil
1 spring onion, trimmed and finely sliced
a large mixed salad, to serve

1. Preheat the oven to 200°C/gas mark 6. Cut 2 large squares
of foil and place on a baking sheet.
2. Divide the courgette, pepper and tomatoes between the foil
sheets and top with the salmon fillets. Place 2 slices of lemon
on each piece of fish, drizzle with the oil and sprinkle with
the spring onion. Bring the foil up around the fish and
vegetables to create two neat parcels. Pinch the edges to seal.
3. Bake in the preheated oven for 20 minutes, until the fish
and vegetables are just cooked. Remove from the oven and
allow to stand for 3 minutes. Open very carefully – the parcels
will be hot. Lift the fish and vegetables on to two plates,
using a spatula. Pour the cooking juices over. Serve with
a large, mixed salad.

Note You can make these parcels up to 12 hours in advance
and keep them in the fridge until you're ready to cook them.
Add 3–4 minutes to the cooking time if you're baking them
straight from chilled.

Beany root vegetable stew

SERVES 4
PREP TIME 10–15 MINS
COOKING TIME 30 MINS

2 tablespoons cold-pressed sunflower oil or extra
    virgin olive oil
1 medium onion, peeled and chopped
8 shallots, peeled
2 celery sticks, trimmed and sliced
4 medium carrots, peeled and sliced
2 medium parsnips or sweet potatoes, peeled and cut
    into roughly 2cm pieces
½ celeriac, peeled and cut into roughly 2cm pieces
    (about 300g prepared weight)
2 garlic cloves, peeled and finely chopped
1 organic vegetable stock cube
750ml just-boiled water
1 tablespoon tomato purée
1 small bay leaf
leaves from a small bunch of fresh thyme (about 1
    tablespoon) or 1 teaspoon dried mixed herbs
2 x 410g tins of mixed beans in water, drained and rinsed
1 tablespoon cornflour, mixed with 2 tablespoons cold
    water to form a smooth paste
freshly chopped flat-leaf parsley, to garnish
lightly cooked shredded Savoy cabbage or green beans,
    to serve

1. Heat the oil in a large saucepan and gently cook the onion,
shallots, celery, carrots, parsnips and celeriac for 10–12
minutes, stirring regularly, until beginning to soften and
very lightly colour without burning. Add the garlic and cook
for about a minute longer.
2. Dissolve the stock cube in the water and pour over the
vegetables. Stir in the tomato purée, bay leaf and thyme or
mixed herbs. Bring to the boil, then reduce the heat, cover
the pan and simmer gently for 15 minutes, stirring
occasionally.

3. Add the beans and cook for 2–3 minutes, until the beans are hot and the vegetables are tender. Stir in the cornflour mixture and cook for 1–2 minutes, stirring regularly, until the sauce thickens. Ladle on to warmed plates and sprinkle with lots of chopped parsley. Serve with freshly cooked cabbage or green beans.

Top tip Chuck a strip of seaweed kombu into any bean dish, as it helps to make beans even more digestible. You don't have to eat it! The minerals from the seaweed will be liberated into the cooking water.

This hearty stew will keep for at least 2 days in the fridge. Reheat in a pan until piping hot, or add a little extra water and blend to a soup before warming through. You can vary the vegetables and beans you use – use a whole celeriac instead of the parsnips, for instance – just keep the quantities roughly the same.

Big time stir

SERVES 2
PREP TIME 10 MINS
COOKING TIME 7 MINS

2 tablespoons olive oil
1 teaspoon sesame oil
2 tablespoons water
½ teaspoon Chinese five-spice
4 spring onions, finely sliced
2 garlic cloves, chopped
1 x 5cm piece of fresh ginger, finely sliced or grated
2 sticks celery, chopped
1 leek, halved and sliced
1 red pepper, chopped (optional)
2 courgettes, sliced
3–4 tablespoons wheat-free tamari soy sauce
1 pok choi, finely sliced
½ Chinese cabbage, finely sliced
125g bag of beansprouts
75g cooked buckwheat noodles
1 bunch of watercress, trimmed
a big bunch of fresh coriander, roughly chopped

1. Place the oils and water in a wok and heat for 1 minute.
Add the five-spice, spring onions, garlic and ginger and cook
for 1 minute, then add the celery, leek, pepper and courgettes
and stir well. Add the tamari and cook for 2–3 minutes.

2. Add the pok choi and Chinese cabbage and cook for 1–2
minutes.

3. Remove from the heat and stir in the beansprouts, noodles
and watercress. Sprinkle with the coriander and serve
immediately.

Chicken and vegetable curry

SERVES 2
PREP TIME 10 MINS
COOKING TIME 18–20 MINS

1 tablespoon cold pressed sunflower oil or extra
   virgin olive oil
1 medium onion, peeled and sliced
150g boneless, skinless chicken breast (preferably
   free-range or organic), cut into roughly 3cm pieces
2 garlic cloves, peeled and crushed
½ teaspoon ground cumin
½ teaspoon ground coriander
½ teaspoon ground turmeric
1 red or orange pepper, deseeded and cut into roughly
   3 cm pieces
150g cauliflower florets (from half a small cauliflower)
75g green beans, trimmed and halved
4 medium tomatoes, quartered
300ml hot vegetable stock (made with an organic
   vegetable stock cube)
50g fresh or frozen peas
2 good handfuls of baby spinach leaves (about 50g)
fresh coriander, to garnish (optional)

1. Heat the oil in a large saucepan and gently cook the onion
and chicken for 2-3 minutes until the chicken is very lightly
coloured on all sides. Add the garlic and spices and cook
together for about a minute to release the flavours.
2. Stir in the pepper, cauliflower, green beans and tomatoes.
Pour over the stock and bring to the boil. Reduce the heat
slightly and simmer gently for 10 minutes, stirring
occasionally.
3. Add the peas and spinach leaves, return to a simmer and
continue cooking for a further 2–3 minutes, until the peas are
just tender and the spinach is wilted. Serve in large bowls,
garnished with plenty of freshly chopped coriander if liked.

Chicken with fresh tomato and pepper salad

SERVES 2
PREP AND COOKING TIME 25 MINS
2 skinless, boneless organic chicken breasts
1 tablespoon olive oil
¼ teaspoon ground cumin, mixed with ¼ teaspoon
   ground coriander
1 tablespoon freshly squeezed lime juice
lightly dressed mixed salad leaves, to serve (optional)

For the tomato and pepper salad

2 large fresh vine tomatoes, roughly chopped
1 small ripe avocado, halved, stoned, peeled and cut into
   roughly 2cm pieces
1 small yellow pepper, halved, deseeded and cut into
   roughly 2 cm pieces
½ small red onion, peeled and finely chopped
1 garlic clove, peeled and crushed
finely grated rind of 1 lime, plus 2 tablespoons lime juice
a small handful of fresh coriander, roughly chopped

1. Toss together all the ingredients for the salad and set
aside. Carefully cut the chicken breasts horizontally almost
all the way through the middle and open out. Brush on both
sides with olive oil and sprinkle with the spices.
2. Pour the remaining oil into a large frying pan or brush over
a griddle and place on a medium heat. When the pan is hot,
add the chicken breasts and cook for 2–3 minutes on each
side until lightly browned and cooked through.
3. Remove the pan from the heat and pour the lime juice over
the chicken. Allow to sizzle for a few seconds. Spoon the salad
on to 2 plates and place the chicken breasts on top. Serve
with a few lightly dressed salad leaves if liked.

Really easy chicken stir-fry

SERVES 2
PREP TIME 8–10 MINS
COOKING TIME 5–6 MINS

1 tablespoon cold pressed sunflower oil
2 small boneless, skinless chicken breasts (preferably
    free-range or organic), thinly sliced
½ red pepper, deseeded and thinly sliced
100g baby corn, trimmed and halved lengthways
freshly squeezed juice of 1 orange (about 5 tablespoons)
1 tablespoon tamari soy sauce
1 teaspoon cornflour or arrowroot powder
100g mangetout, trimmed
1 green pok choi (about 125g), washed and thickly shredded
1 garlic clove, peeled and finely chopped or crushed
2 spring onions, trimmed and sliced
fresh beansprouts and chopped cashew nuts (optional)

1. Heat a large non-stick frying pan or wok. Add the oil,
½ teaspoon water and then the chicken strips. Stir-fry over
a medium heat for 1–2 minutes, until lightly coloured. Add
the pepper and baby corn and cook for 2 minutes. Blend the
orange juice, tamari and cornflour in a small bowl; set aside.
2. Add the mangetout and pok choi to the chicken and
vegetable mixture and continue stir-frying for a further
minute until the chicken is cooked through. Then add the
garlic and spring onions. Stir-fry for about 30 seconds,
then pour over the cornflour mixture.
3. Cook until the sauce thickens, becomes glossy and lightly
coats the chicken and vegetables. Remove from the heat and
serve on warmed plates or in deep bowls. Top with lots of
crunchy beansprouts and sprinkle with a few finely chopped
plain cashew nuts if you like.

Note Stir a little Chinese five-spice powder in with the
garlic and spring onions for a more intense flavour.

Grilled sea bass with herb sauce

SERVES 2
PREP TIME 8 MINS
COOKING TIME 8 MINS

2 x 150g sea bass fillets
1 teaspoon extra virgin olive oil

For the herb sauce

2 tablespoons finely chopped fresh parsley
1 tablespoon finely chopped fresh tarragon
1 tablespoon finely chopped fresh young thyme leaves
4 tablespoons extra virgin olive oil
1 teaspoon cider vinegar
1 garlic clove, peeled and finely chopped
1 teaspoon Dijon mustard

1. Mix all the ingredients for the herb sauce in a small bowl and set aside. Place the fish fillets, skin side up, on a grill pan lined with well-oiled foil.
2. Brush the skin with a little more oil and cook the fish under a hot preheated grill for 5–7 minutes or until the skin is beginning to crisp and the fish is cooked through. (The skin will protect the fish and keep it wonderfully moist – you can tell when the fish is cooked, because it will have turned white.)
3. Transfer to 2 warmed plates, turning the fish over very gently with a spatula. Spoon over the herb sauce. Serve with plenty of lightly cooked vegetables such as green beans, baby carrots and mangetout.

Marinated tofu with lemon sauce

Prepare the tofu first and then make the sauce.

SERVES 2
PREP AND COOKING TIME 25 MINS
1 x 250g packs of firm pressed tofu

For the marinade

1 tablespoon agave syrup
2 teaspoons toasted sesame oil
2 teaspoons wheat-free tamari soy sauce
1 teaspoon mirin
2 teaspoons sesame seeds
2 tablespoons finely chopped fresh coriander

1. Drain the tofu and gently squeeze out as much water as you can with your hands.
2. Place on a clean chopping board between two layers of double thickness kitchen roll and press out any remaining liquid.
3. Cut in half horizontally so that you have 2 squares approximately 1cm thick. Cut these into quarters.
4. Mix the marinade together in a shallow dish and add the tofu squares, coating each side in marinade. Be gentle with handling the tofu, as it can easily break. Cover and chill in the fridge for 2–4 hours. Drain well in a colander.
5. This can be eaten cold and raw or grilled. Serve with steamed pok choi or a crunchy salad. Any excess marinade can be thinned with a little water and drizzled over the pok choi or salad.

For the lemon sauce

**5 thin strips unwaxed lemon zest (use a potato peeler
   to remove the strips)**
2 tablespoons finely shredded fresh root ginger
200ml cold water
4 teaspoons light agave syrup
1 teaspoon organic vegetable bouillon (stock) powder
2 teaspoons cornflour
2 tablespoons wheat-free tamari soy sauce
freshly squeezed juice of half a lemon

1. Put the lemon zest, ginger, water, agave syrup and
bouillon in a small pan. Bring to the boil, stirring constantly.
Mix together the cornflour, tamari and lemon juice in a
small dish and add to the pan, stirring until it thickens.
2. Serve over the tofu.

Mediterranean-style cod stew

SERVES 2
PREP AND COOKING TIME 35–40 MINS
1 tablespoon extra virgin olive oil
1 medium onion, peeled and finely sliced
2 garlic cloves, peeled and sliced
½ teaspoon fennel seeds (optional)
1 x 400g tin of chopped tomatoes
200ml just-boiled water
a good pinch of saffron threads
1 teaspoon dried mixed herbs
1 teaspoon organic vegetable bouillon (stock) powder
1 courgette, trimmed and cut into 1cm slices
300g thick cod fillet, skinned and cut into roughly 4cm pieces

1. Heat the oil in a large saucepan and gently sweat the onion for 3 minutes until beginning to soften. Add the garlic and fennel seeds and cook for 2 minutes more, stirring regularly.
2. Tip the tomatoes into the pan and add the water, saffron, mixed herbs and stock powder. Bring to the boil, then reduce the heat and leave to simmer for 10 minutes, adding the courgette after 5 minutes. Stir occasionally.
3. Scatter the fish over the top of the simmering stew and leave to cook gently for 4–5 minutes, without stirring. Serve with lots of freshly cooked green vegetables.

Mung stew

MAKES 4 SERVINGS (SAVE SOME FOR NEXT DAY'S
LUNCH OR DINNER)
PREP TIME 15 MINS
COOKING TIME 25 MINS

1 tablespoon extra virgin olive oil
1 medium onion, peeled and chopped
2 garlic cloves, peeled and finely chopped
3 medium carrots, peeled and cut into roughly 1cm slices
3 celery sticks, trimmed and cut into roughly 1cm slices
150g dried mung beans, rinsed
1.75 litres just-boiled water
1 organic vegetable stock cube
2 tablespoons tomato purée
2 teaspoons dried mixed herbs or 2 tablespoons finely
    chopped fresh mixed herbs
2 leeks, trimmed and cut into roughly 0.5cm slices
100g roughly shredded curly kale or Savoy cabbage
2 teaspoons cornflour, mixed with 1 tablespoon cold
    water to form a smooth paste

1. Heat the oil in a large saucepan or flameproof casserole
and gently fry the onion for 3 minutes, stirring regularly.
Add the garlic and cook for 2 minutes more, until softened
but not coloured.
2. Add the carrots and celery and continue cooking for
3–4 minutes, or until beginning to soften. Stir in the mung
beans, water, stock cube, tomato purée and herbs. Bring to
the boil, then reduce the heat slightly and simmer gently
for 25 minutes, stirring occasionally.
3. Add the leeks and kale and cook for 5 minutes more,
adding more water if necessary. When the mung beans are
tender, stir in the cornflour mixture and heat until the sauce
is thickened and glossy, stirring regularly. Serve with freshly
boiled brown rice if liked.

Scrumptious stuffed peppers

SERVES 2
PREP TIME 10 MINS
COOKING TIME 50 MINS

1 medium red onion, peeled and cut into eighths
1 medium courgette, trimmed and cut into roughly 1cm slices
1 medium sweet potato, peeled and cut into roughly 2cm
    chunks
2 tablespoons extra virgin olive oil, plus a little extra for
    drizzling
2 medium red peppers, halved lengthways and deseeded
50g quinoa, rinsed
25g pine nuts
1 teaspoon organic vegetable bouillon (stock) powder
1½ teaspoons dried mixed herbs, or 2 tablespoons
    chopped fresh mixed herbs

1. Preheat the oven to 200°C/gas mark 6. Toss the onion,
courgette and sweet potato with 1 tablespoon of the oil
and tip on to a large baking tray. Bake for 25 minutes.
2. Remove the tray and turn all the vegetables. Add the
pepper halves to the tray, cut side down. Return to the oven
for a further 10 minutes or until the vegetables are tender
and lightly browned.
3. While the vegetables are roasting, cook the quinoa in
boiling water for 10–12 minutes until tender, then drain in
a sieve under running water until cold. Tip into a large bowl.
Add the chopped roasted vegetables and stir in the remaining
olive oil, pine nuts, stock powder and herbs until well mixed.
4. Place the pepper halves, cut side up, on the baking tray.
Fill the pepper halves with the quinoa mixture, drizzle with a
little more oil and return to the oven for a further 15 minutes,
or until the peppers are just tender. Serve with lots of lightly
dressed raw salad.

MAIN SALADS

Aduki beans with red onion and corn salsa

Aduki beans are now available in cans from all health food stores and large supermarkets. For a change, you can substitute black-eyed peas. This dish makes a great salad salsa on its own, or can be served with oily fish such as salmon or mackerel. It also makes a great snack or quick lunch. Add a little hemp oil to taste, as an option.

SERVES 2
PREP TIME 2–3 MINS – THE TIME IT TAKES TO OPEN 2 CANS
AND CHOP AN ONION
1 x 400g tin of aduki beans, drained (175g drained weight)
80g organic sweetcorn
75g red onion, finely chopped
2 tablespoons cider vinegar
a handful of fresh parsley, chopped

1. Mix all the ingredients together and serve.

Crunchy walnut coleslaw

SERVES 4–6
PREP TIME 10 MINS

½ red or white cabbage, cored and finely shredded
4 medium carrots, peeled and grated
2 celery sticks, trimmed and sliced
1 red pepper, deseeded and sliced
50g fresh peas (weight after podding)
3 spring onions, trimmed and sliced
100g walnut halves or pumpkin seeds
1 tablespoon chopped fresh parsley (optional)

For the dressing

3 tablespoons extra virgin olive oil
1 tablespoon cider vinegar
½ teaspoon Dijon mustard
½ garlic clove, peeled and crushed (optional)

1. Place all the salad ingredients, except the nuts or seeds, in a large bowl. Place the dressing ingredients in a jug with 3 tablespoons cold water and blend with a stick blender until thick (alternatively whisk with a fork). Fold into the salad. Cover and chill until ready to serve. Sprinkle with nuts or seeds just before serving.

Note This salad is perfect for lunchboxes and can be made the night before. Add the nuts or seeds just before you leave the house, so they remain crunchy.

Easy peasy pea salad

SERVES 2
PREP TIME 5 MINS
300g tin of black-eyed peas
175g frozen peas
10 silverskin onions
3–4 tablespoons cider vinegar
2 tablespoons olive oil
a handful of fresh mint, chopped

1. Drain the black-eyed peas and place them in a bowl.
Pour the frozen peas into the empty tin to measure an
equal amount and add to the bowl.

2. Add the onions, vinegar, olive oil and mint.

3. Stir well and leave for 2 minutes for the peas to defrost.
You can also use fresh peas.

4. This salad keeps well in the fridge for 1 day.

Fatoush

I make my fatoush with butter beans, which gives a great texture. You can use borlotti beans too.

SERVES 2
PREP TIME 5 MINS
COOKING TIME 5 MINS

1 tablespoon sesame seeds
400g tin of butter beans or borlotti beans, drained and rinsed
1 cucumber, halved, seeds scooped out, sliced
4 spring onions, sliced
2 handfuls fresh parsley, chopped
1 handful fresh mint leaves, chopped
1 tablespoon capers, drained
3 tablespoons olive oil
Juice of 2 lemons

1. Place the sesame seeds in a non-stick pan and cook over a moderate heat for a couple of minutes, until golden in colour.
2. Mix all the other ingredients together and sprinkle with the sesame seeds.

Note It's great to serve this on a bed of coriander and rocket, or with some sprouted alfalfalfa seeds and pok choi. And add brown rice to turn fatoush into a main meal.

Layered Mexican salad

SERVES 2
PREP TIME 7 MINS
100g mixed salad leaves
4 large tomatoes
4 spring onions, chopped
1 x 400g tin of red kidney beans, drained and rinsed
1 small tin of organic corn drained
2 tablespoons cider vinegar
6 tablespoons olive oil
a handful of fresh coriander, chopped
1 ripe avocado
2 tablespoons lemon juice

1. Place the salad leaves in the bottom of a glass bowl
or deep pie dish.

2. Dice the tomatoes, mix with the onion and add to the
leaves, then add a layer of beans and another of corn. Mix
the vinegar and oil together with a tablespoon of the chopped
coriander and pour over the salad; this can all be done in
advance.

3. Chop the avocado and mix with the lemon juice. Scatter
over the salad with the remaining coriander, and serve
immediately.

Lentil salad

SERVES 2 (AND LEAVES YOU WITH EXTRA FOR
A SIDE DISH OR SNACK)
PREP TIME 7 MINS
COOKING TIME 12 MINS

100g red lentils
4 shallots
2 garlic cloves
1 generous teaspoon chopped fresh ginger
2 generous teaspoons wheat-free vegetable bouillon
   (stock) powder
100g fresh rocket
2 tablespoons chopped fresh coriander
4 lime wedges

1. Rinse and drain the lentils. Place in a medium-sized saucepan.

2. Add the shallots, garlic, ginger and bouillon powder and cover with cold water. Bring to the boil, then lower heat and simmer for 12 minutes, stirring now and again.

3. Remove from the heat and drain away any excess water.

4. Divide the rocket between serving plates and pile the lentils on top.

5. Garnish with coriander and lime wedges, and serve.

Moroccan chickpea salad

SERVES 2 AS A MAIN COURSE OR 4 AS A SIDE DISH
PREP TIME 10 MINS
COOKING TIME 30 MINS

100g brown rice
2 tablespoons olive oil
2 tablespoons water
1 medium onion, sliced
1 leek, sliced
1 garlic clove, crushed
1 teaspoon ground cumin
½ teaspoon ground coriander
¼ teaspoon ground cinnamon
1 x 400g tin of chickpeas, drained and rinsed in cold water
50g frozen peas
juice of 1 lemon
2 tablespoons freshly chopped coriander
50g baby spinach leaves

1. Place the rice in a medium-sized pan of cold water and bring to the boil. Cover and allow to simmer for 20–25 minutes, or until tender.

2. Meanwhile heat the oil and water in a medium-sized frying pan, add the onion and leek and cook gently for 3 minutes. Stir in the garlic and spices and cook for 2 minutes, stirring regularly. Remove from the heat and allow to cool.

3. Drain the cooked rice and rinse in cold water.

4. Transfer the rice to a large bowl and add the spiced onion mixture, the chickpeas, peas, lemon juice and coriander.

5. Arrange the spinach leaves on a serving plate and top with the salad.

Note This can be made in advance and will keep well for 2–3 days, covered, in the fridge.

Buckwheat noodle salad with pok choi and sesame dressing

SERVES 2
PREP TIME 12 MINS
COOKING TIME 3–5 MINS

150g buckwheat noodles
2 tablespoons wheat-free tamari soy sauce
1 tablespoon cider vinegar
2 tablespoons olive oil
1 dessertspoon white miso
a few drops of sesame oil
2 pok choi (200g), white part finely sliced, green leaves
    left whole
a handful of sprouting beans
sunflower or sesame seeds to garnish

1. Bring a pan of water to the boil and add the noodles.
Cook for 2–3 minutes, according to preference, then strain
into a colander and rinse with plenty of cold water.

2. Combine the tamari, vinegar, olive oil, white miso and
sesame oil in a bowl and whisk to combine.

3. Steam the green leaves of the pok choi for 1–2 minutes,
until just wilted – do not overcook.

4. Add the noodles to the dressing with all the pok choi
and stir well.

5. Transfer to 2 serving bowls and garnish with the
sprouting beans and sunflower or sesame seeds.

Nori sushi rolls with dipping sauce

SERVES 2
PREP TIME 15 MINS

2 small ripe avocados, halved, stoned, peeled
  and roughly chopped
2 spring onions
½ garlic clove, peeled
¼ teaspoon ground coriander
freshly squeezed juice of 1 lime or ½ lemon
1 pack of nori sheets (4 sheets in each pack)
pickled ginger

Vegetable fillings

a selection of different fillings in separate bowls
  – e.g. peeled and finely grated carrots, alfalfa
  or mung beansprouts, finely shredded Savoy
  cabbage or Chinese leaf, thin sticks of cucumber
  and cooked brown rice – about 1 cup of each
2–3 tablespoons chopped fresh dill or parsley

Soy dipping sauce

1 tablespoon wheat-free tamari soy sauce
1 tablespoon water
½ garlic clove, peeled and sliced (optional)
sliced spring onion and a little finely diced red
  pepper, to garnish

1. Place the avocados, onions, garlic, coriander and lemon
or lime juice in a food processor or liquidizer and blend until
smooth (you can also use a stick blender for this job).
2. Place a sheet of nori, shiny side down, on a board. (Do not
rinse the nori. It is the one seaweed that does not need to be
rinsed.) Spread with a quarter of the avocado mixture,
leaving a large gap at the top. If you put too much on, the
spread will start to ooze out at the sides and the nori may
become a little soggy. The more you do this, the better you
will get at knowing how much spread is needed. Place narrow

rows of raw vegetables, starting from the bottom of the nori, across roughly half the sheet. Sprinkle with the dill and add some pickled ginger.

3. Roll up the nori from the bottom, squeezing tightly to hold the filling. When rolled it should be firm and strong. Cut into 4–5 rolls with a very sharp knife and put on a serving plate. Repeat the method using the remaining nori, avocado paste and fillings.

4. Mix all the ingredients for the dipping sauce in a small bowl and serve with the sushi.

Note If you don't have a liquidizer or food processor, you can chop the onions and garlic finely, add to the other ingredients and mash really well with a potato masher. Or simply use well-mashed plain avocado for the filling paste. Nori sushi rolls make a fantastic snack too.

Quinoa and mixed bean salad

SERVES 4
PREP TIME 15 MINS
COOKING TIME 10 MINS

75g quinoa
2 teaspoons bouillon powder
100g frozen broad beans, thawed
50g fresh peas
1 x 420g tin of mixed beans in water, drained and rinsed
2 celery sticks, trimmed and sliced
3 tablespoons pumpkin seeds
2 spring onions, trimmed and finely sliced, or ¼ red onion,
    peeled and finely sliced
a small handful of fresh mint leaves, roughly chopped
a small handful of fresh parsley leaves, roughly chopped
2 tablespoons virgin olive oil
1 teaspoon cider vinegar
1 garlic clove, peeled and crushed
juice from ½ small lemon

1. Bring a medium pan of water to the boil. Stir in the
bouillon powder and quinoa. Boil for about 10 minutes until
the quinoa is tender. Drain in a sieve, then rinse under
running water until cold. Press the quinoa with the back
of a spoon to remove the excess water, then tip it into a
serving bowl.
2. Slip the broad beans out of their skins and add the tender
inner part of each bean to the quinoa. Stir in the peas, tinned
beans, celery, pumpkin seeds, spring onions, mint, parsley,
oil, vinegar and garlic. Toss well together. Stand for at least
20 minutes before serving to allow the flavours to develop.
Season with fresh lemon juice to taste and serve.

Top tip This salad keeps well for 1–2 days and makes a great
packed lunch, full of fibre and flavour. Serve as a filling salad
after vegetable or miso soup, on a bed of crisp salad leaves,
or spoon into baked sweet potatoes.

Tomato, avocado and red onion salad with basil dressing

SERVES 2
PREP TIME 10 MINS

3 medium-large vine tomatoes, sliced
½ small red onion, peeled and finely sliced
1 small ripe avocado, halved, stoned, sliced and peeled
a good handful of fresh basil leaves
50g pitted olives, drained
2 tablespoons pine nuts

For the dressing

1 tablespoon extra virgin olive oil
1 tablespoon cold-pressed sunflower oil
1 teaspoon organic cider vinegar
6 large basil leaves

1. To make the dressing, place all the ingredients in a jug and blend with a stick blender until smooth.

2. Arrange the tomatoes, onion, avocado and basil leaves in a shallow serving dish and scatter the olives and pine nuts over. Drizzle with the basil dressing just before serving.

Note If you don't have a stick blender, chop the basil leaves finely and whisk into the other ingredients until the dressing is well mixed.

Very easy tuna salad

SERVES 2
PREP TIME 7 MINS

a small bag of watercress, rocket and spinach salad
1 x 200g tin of tuna in spring water, drained
75g cucumber, sliced
8 cherry tomatoes, halved
a small handful of mixed olives in olive oil, drained
   (optional)
2 tablespoons extra virgin olive oil
1 teaspoon good quality balsamic vinegar

1. Share the salad leaves over 2 plates. Divide the tuna between the salads.

2. Add the cucumber, tomatoes and olives, if using.

3. Drizzle with olive oil and vinegar, and serve.

Warm chicken salad

SERVES 1
PREP TIME 10 MINS
COOKING TIME 15–20 MINS
1 boneless, skinless organic chicken breast
75g green beans
75g asparagus spears
2 tablespoons pine nuts
6 halved cherry tomatoes
a handful of basil leaves
a bag of baby leaf salad

For the dressing

2 teaspoons olive oil
1 teaspoon cider vinegar
½ teaspoon Dijon mustard
1 tablespoon water

1. Place the chicken breast in a medium pan and cover with 200ml of water.
2. Bring to the boil, cover with a lid and simmer for 15–20 minutes, until the chicken is cooked (alternatively, cook in a steamer according to the manufacturer's instructions.)
3. Meanwhile, steam the beans and asparagus lightly.
4. Remove the chicken from the pan and place it on a board. Leave it for 2–3 minutes, then slice it thinly and toss it in a bowl with the beans, asparagus, pine nuts, tomatoes, basil leaves and some baby leaf salad.
5. Mix together the ingredients for the dressing and drizzle over the salad. Serve while the chicken is still warm.

VEGETABLES AND SIDES

Avocado, tomato and basil side salad

SERVES 2
PREP TIME 10 MINS
2 ripe avocados, halved
4 vine-ripened tomatoes, sliced
2 handfuls of fresh basil leaves
15g pine nuts
2 tablespoons extra virgin olive oil
1 teaspoon good-quality balsamic vinegar

1. Stone the avocados and slice thickly. Peel off the skin and discard.
2. Arrange the avocado slices on 2 serving plates and top with the tomatoes and basil leaves. Sprinkle with pine nuts.
3. Drizzle with olive oil and balsamic vinegar to serve.

Cabbage and fennel with lemon and thyme

SERVES 2
PREP TIME 7 MINS
500g white cabbage, cored and finely shredded
2 fennel bulbs, cored and finely shredded
juice of 2 lemons
6 tablespoons olive oil
1 teaspoon fresh thyme leaves
1 teaspoon dried fennel seeds
1 tablespoon fresh parsley

1. Toss all the ingredients together in a large bowl and serve.

Celeriac and carrot purée

SERVES 2–3
PREP TIME 10 MINS
COOKING TIME 12–15 MINS
1 medium celeriac
3 medium carrots, peeled and thinly sliced
1 teaspoon organic vegetable bouillon (stock) powder
1 tablespoon freshly snipped chives, to garnish (optional)

1. Peel the celeriac and cut into roughly 3cm pieces. Put it into a saucepan with the carrots and cover with plenty of cold water. Bring to the boil and cook for 12–15 minutes, or until the vegetables are very tender.
2. Drain in a colander, then return to the saucepan and sprinkle with the stock powder. Either mash or purée with a stick blender until smooth. Warm through gently before serving, and sprinkle with fresh chives if liked.

Cooling salad

SERVES 2
PREP TIME 10 MINS
250g fresh peas, washed
100g mangetout, trimmed and halved lengthways
4 spring onions, trimmed and sliced
½ cucumber, trimmed and cut into roughly 2cm pieces
a small handful of freshly shredded mint leaves
2 tablespoons freshly snipped chives
4 tablespoons natural soya yogurt
1 garlic clove, peeled and crushed

1. Toss all the ingredients together lightly and tip into a serving dish. Cover and chill for 30–60 minutes before serving.

Crunchy courgette and carrot salad

SERVES 4 AS A SIDE DISH AND 2 AS A MAIN MEAL SALAD
PREP TIME 10 MINS

100g white cabbage, finely shredded
2 medium carrots, peeled and thinly sliced diagonally
½ red pepper, deseeded and finely sliced
1 medium courgette, trimmed and finely sliced
¼ medium onion, peeled and finely chopped
2 tablespoons pumpkin or sunflower seeds
2 tablespoons pine nuts
1 tablespoon freshly squeezed lemon juice
5 tablespoons plain soya yogurt

1. Toss the cabbage, carrots, pepper, courgette, onion, pumpkin seeds and pine nuts together.
2. Drizzle with lemon juice, spoon over the soya yogurt, toss well and serve.

Green beans with warm cherry tomatoes and garlic

SERVES 2
COOKING TIME 12 MINS
150g fine green beans, trimmed
2 teaspoons extra virgin olive oil
½ small onion, halved and chopped
2 garlic cloves, peeled and finely sliced
100g ripe cherry plum tomatoes, halved

1. Cook the beans in a pan of boiling water for 5–7 minutes, until tender. Meanwhile, heat the oil in a small frying pan and gently fry the onion and garlic for 4–5 minutes, stirring regularly until softened.
2. Add the tomatoes and continue cooking for a further 2 minutes, until they have softened but still retain their shape.
3. Drain the beans, then return them to the saucepan and add the tomato and onion. Toss well together and serve.

Millet mash and onion gravy

SERVES 4
PREP TIME 10 MINS
COOKING TIME 25–30 MINS

100g millet
herbal seasoning or a pinch of sea salt
1 onion, peeled and chopped
1 cauliflower, cut into small florets
Onion gravy (see below)

1. Wash the millet and drain. Put it into a medium-sized pan, add the seasoning and bring to the boil. Simmer for 20 minutes.

2. Meanwhile place the onion and cauliflower in a second pan and cover with water. Bring to the boil, then lower the heat and simmer for 5 minutes. Remove from the heat, drain and return to the pan. Mash with a potato masher.

3. Drain the millet and mix into the mashed cauliflower and onion mixture. Serve warm, with the onion gravy.

For the onion gravy

MAKES 250ML
COOKING TIME 25–30 MINS

2 onions, peeled and sliced
2 teaspoons olive oil
2 teaspoons tamari soy sauce
2 teaspoons arrowroot

1. Place the onion and olive oil in a pan with 6 tablespoons of water and cook gently for 15–20 minutes, until the onions are translucent.

2. Mix the tamari with the arrowroot and add to the onion mixture along with 500ml of just-boiled water, mixing well.

3. Cook over a medium heat for 10 minutes and serve hot.

Mixed leaves with Brazil nut pesto

SERVES 2
PREP TIME 5 MINS

200g mixed salad leaves, e.g. watercress, rocket,
    radicchio, baby spinach or chard
3 sticks celery, sliced
leaves of 1 Belgian endive
a handful of mixed sprouting beans

For the pesto

175g whole Brazil nuts
200ml olive oil
3 garlic cloves, peeled
a large handful of coriander leaves (about 60g)
juice of 2 lemons

1. Place all the ingredients for the pesto in a food processor
or blender and process until smooth.

2. Place the salad leaves in a bowl with the celery and endive,
add the pesto and toss to coat the leaves.

3. Sprinkle over the sprouting beans and serve immediately.

Roasted vegetables with pine nuts

PREP TIME 15 MINS
COOKING TIME 45 MINS

A selection of vegetables – sweet potatoes, red peppers, courgettes, red onion wedges and garlic cloves – are drizzled with olive oil and roasted in the oven until golden. Pine nuts and cherry tomatoes are added for the last 10 minutes of cooking time. Serve with a fresh raw salad. (Leftover roasted vegetables can be served cold in a quinoa salad for next day's lunch.)

Note This can be a main meal or a vegetable side.

Savoury vegetable rice

SERVES 2
PREP AND COOKING TIME 40 MINS
150g brown rice, rinsed
2 teaspoons organic vegetable bouillon (stock) powder
1 tablespoon extra virgin olive oil
½ medium red onion, peeled and chopped
1 medium carrot, peeled and finely sliced
½ red pepper, deseeded and cut into roughly 1.5 cm pieces
1 garlic clove, peeled and finely chopped
1 medium courgette, trimmed and cut into roughly
    1.5cm cubes
50g frozen peas
nori (seaweed) flakes (optional)

1. Cook the rice with the stock powder in boiling water for
25–30 minutes, or according to the packet instructions.
2. While the rice is cooking, heat the oil in a large frying pan
and gently fry the onion, carrot and pepper for 5 minutes,
until softened.
3. Add the garlic and courgette and cook for 2 minutes more,
then stir in the peas. Cook over a very gentle heat until the
peas are hot, stirring regularly.
4. Drain the rice and tip into the pan with the vegetables.
Toss together well and serve, sprinkled with nori flakes if
you like.

Spinach and tofu with mixed leaves and watercress dressing

SERVES 2
PREP AND COOKING TIME 5 MINS
200g baby spinach leaves
200g tofu
100g baby salad leaves
2 garlic cloves
100g watercress
2 tablespoons cider vinegar
1 tablespoon wheat-free tamari soy sauce
8 tablespoons olive oil
dried seaweed to garnish

1. Lightly steam the spinach for 1–2 minutes, then arrange on plates with the tofu (see page 172 for how to prepare) and salad leaves.

2. Place the garlic, watercress, vinegar, tamari and olive oil in a food processor or blender and process until smooth. Pour this dressing over the salad, sprinkle over the seaweed and serve.

Sprouting salad

SERVES 1
PREP TIME 10 MINS
125g cucumber, finely sliced
25g bean sprouts
25g alfalfa sprouts
30g fresh watercress leaves
juice of ½ lemon
2 tablespoons chopped fresh mint
a couple of pok choi leaves
1 generous tablespoon of shelled hemp seeds
6 water chestnuts (optional)

1. Mix the cucumber, sprouts, watercress, lemon juice and mint in a bowl. Add the pok choi leaves and sprinkle with shelled hemp seeds. Add water chestnuts for a crunchy texture.

Steamed cabbage with sesame cashew nuts

SERVES 2
PREP TIME 5 MINS
COOKING TIME 5 MINS
500g white or green cabbage, cored and shredded
1 teaspoon sesame oil
1 tablespoon water
100g cashew nuts
1 tablespoon wheat-free tamari soy sauce

1. Steam the cabbage for just 3 minutes so that it is still crisp and green.

2. Meanwhile place the sesame oil and water in a non-stick frying pan and cook over a high heat for about 1–2 minutes, until the water boils and evaporates.

3. Add the cashew nuts and tamari followed by the steamed cabbage, stir well and serve immediately.

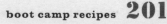

Sunrise salad

½ fennel bulb, trimmed and finely sliced
14 radishes, trimmed and halved
2 medium carrots, peeled and thinly sliced diagonally
40g plain unsalted cashew nuts
2 tablespoons sunflower seeds
2 tablespoons pumpkin seeds
1 punnet of freshly snipped cress

For the dressing

2 tablespoons freshly squeezed orange juice
1 tablespoon extra virgin olive oil
¼ teaspoon sesame oil
½ garlic clove, peeled and crushed
½ teaspoon wholegrain mustard

1. Whisk the orange juice, oils, garlic and mustard together to make the dressing, and set aside.
2. Gently toss the fennel, radishes, carrots, nuts, sunflower and pumpkin seeds. Spoon over the dressing, sprinkle with cress and serve.

Sweet and sour vegetables

SERVES 2
PREP TIME 7 MINS
COOKING TIME 8 MINS

1 tablespoon cold-pressed sunflower oil
2 medium carrots, peeled and sliced
1 medium-large courgette, trimmed and sliced
½ red pepper, deseeded and cut into roughly 2cm pieces
150g small broccoli florets
100g baby corn, trimmed and halved lengthways
3 spring onions, trimmed and sliced
2 garlic cloves, peeled and crushed
1 teaspoon finely grated fresh ginger
50g plain cashew nuts (optional)
1 teaspoon cornflour, blended with 1 tablespoon cold water
1 tablespoon organic cider vinegar
1 teaspoon tomato purée
1 tablespoon light agave syrup
4 tablespoons cold water

1. Heat the oil in a large frying pan or wok and stir-fry the carrots, courgettes, red pepper, broccoli and baby corn for 4–5 minutes.

2. Add the spring onions, garlic and ginger, and the cashew nuts, if using, and cook for a further minute, stirring. Mix the cornflour paste, vinegar, tomato purée, agave syrup and cold water.

3. Stir into the pan and cook for 1 minute more, until the sauce is glossy and lightly coats all the vegetables. Serve.

White bean mash

SERVES 2
PREP TIME 6 MINS
COOKING TIME 7 MINS

1 x 410g tin of butter beans, drained
½ tablespoon white miso
60ml vegetable stock
2 tablespoons olive oil
3 spring onions, chopped
fresh chopped chives
fresh chopped parsley to garnish

1. Place the butter beans, white miso and stock in the food processor with 1 tablespoon of olive oil and blend until smooth.
2. Place the remaining oil in a small pan with 1 tablespoon of water, add the onions and cook over a moderate heat for 3–4 minutes. Add the butter bean mixture and cook, stirring constantly, for 2–3 minutes.
3. Remove from the heat, stir in the chives, and serve immediately, garnished with parsley.

SNACKS

Avocado stuffed with black-eyed peas

SERVES 4
PREP TIME 5 MINS

2 avocados, halved, stone removed
a squeeze of lemon juice
1 x 300g tin of black-eyed peas, drained
200g cherry tomatoes, halved
2 spring onions, chopped
1 tablespoon cider vinegar
2 tablespoons fresh basil

1. Place the avocado halves on 4 serving plates and sprinkle over the lemon juice.
2. Mix all the other ingredients together, spoon into the avocados and serve immediately.

Avocado vinaigrette

SERVES 2
PREP TIME 5 MINS
1 large ripe avocado
mixed salad leaves, to garnish (optional)

For the dressing

2 tablespoons extra virgin olive oil
1 tablespoon cold-pressed sunflower oil
1 tablespoon organic cider vinegar
1 teaspoon Dijon mustard
1 teaspoon agave syrup
1 small garlic clove, peeled and crushed (optional)

1. To make the dressing, put all the vinaigrette ingredients in a bowl and whisk together until thickened and glossy.
2. Cut the avocado in half and remove the stone. Put the avocado halves on 2 small plates and garnish with salad leaves if liked. Pour the dressing into the avocados and serve.

Herby nuts

MAKES 6 SERVINGS
PREP AND COOKING TIME 10 MINS
200g mixed plain nuts, such as Brazils, pistachios,
   cashews, almonds and hazelnuts
1 tablespoon extra virgin olive oil
1 tablespoon chopped fresh rosemary
1 tablespoon chopped fresh thyme leaves
a dash of tamari soy sauce (optional)

1. Preheat the oven to 190°C/gas mark 5. Put the nuts into
a bowl and toss with the olive oil, herbs and tamari sauce
if using. Tip on to a shallow baking tray.

2. Bake for 5 minutes, then carefully remove the tray from
the oven and turn the nuts. Return to the oven for a further
2–3 minutes, until the nuts are warm and the herbs are
fragrant – do not allow the nuts to turn brown.

3. Serve the nuts just warm as a snack, or leave them to cool
and store them in an airtight jar for up to 3 days. Good for
sprinkling over salads.

Lemon and coriander hummus

MAKES 6 SERVINGS
PREP TIME 10 MINS
1 x 410g tin of chickpeas, drained and rinsed
3 tablespoons light tahini
finely grated zest of ½ small lemon
freshly squeezed juice of 1 small lemon
1 teaspoon organic vegetable bouillon (stock) powder
3 tablespoons extra virgin olive oil
4 tablespoons cold water
3 tablespoons finely chopped fresh coriander leaves

1. Put all the ingredients except the coriander into a food processor and blend until smooth – you may have to remove the lid and push the mixture down a couple of times with a rubber spatula until you have the right consistency.
2. Remove the blade and stir in the coriander – add a little more lemon juice to taste if liked. Spoon into a bowl and serve with plenty of fresh vegetable sticks for dipping.

Olive tapenade

PREP TIME 5 MINS
100g pitted black olives
2 garlic cloves, peeled and crushed
1 teaspoon lemon juice

1. Blend all the ingredients until smooth. Store in a jar in the fridge.

Convenient snacks

» Any piece of fruit

» Dried goji berries

» Pomegranate seeds

» Any vegetable

» Vegetable crudités with dips, pâtés or spreads

» Dates

» Nuts, salt free: almonds, cashews, hazelnuts, pine nuts, pecans, walnuts, Brazil and macadamia nuts

» Chestnuts: they come in glass jars or vacuum-packed (eat as they are, or warm in the oven for 10 minutes)

» Seeds: raw shelled hemp, flax, sunflower, pumpkin

» Toasted nori (seaweed) strips (available in health food stores)

» Sprouted chickpeas (leave some dried chickpeas in a bowl of water for 24–48 hours – they will start to sprout, and you have a tasty chewy snack

» Mashed avocado (you can mix it with hummus too)

» Fruit and nut bars, but make sure they are free of chemicals and cane sugar

» Oatcakes with nut butter

» Tabbouleh

TREATS

Baked apples with prunes and walnuts

SERVES 4
PREP TIME 10 MINS
COOKING TIME 35 MINS
25g sultanas
25g raisins
6 pitted prunes, chopped
25g walnut halves, chopped
½ teaspoon ground mixed spice
1 tablespoon light agave syrup
4 medium Bramley cooking apples
1 teaspoon sunflower oil, for greasing

1. Preheat the oven to 180°C/gas mark 4. Mix together the sultanas, raisins, prunes, walnuts, spice and agave syrup.

2. Core the apples, using an apple corer through the centre and creating a hole at least 3cm in diameter. Score through the skin around the equator of each apple. Place in a lightly oiled baking dish.

3. Fill the apples with the fruit mixture. Bake in the centre of the preheated oven for 35 minutes, or until the apples are soft, and serve.

Note These apples are also delicious cold: simply slip off the skins and mash the softened apples roughly with the dried fruits.

Mango and pineapple jelly

There are a number of really good natural juices that are additive free, available in supermarkets and health shops. Agar flakes are available from supermarkets and health food shops and are really easy to use.

SERVES 2
PREP TIME 10 MINUTES, PLUS CHILLING TIME
1 tablespoon agar flakes
250ml natural pineapple juice
1 ripe mango (300g), peeled, stoned and cubed

1. Place the agar flakes and juice in a small pan and stir well. Place over a moderate heat and cook until the agar has dissolved, then bring to the boil, allow to boil for 2–3 minutes and remove from the heat.
2. Leave to cool for 5 minutes, then stir in the mango. Pour into a 300–400ml mould or bowl and chill for 1–2 hours, until set.

Spiced rice pudding

SERVES 2–3
COOKING TIME 35 MINS
25g pudding rice
50g brown rice, rinsed
600–800ml rice milk
6 cardamom pods
1 cinnamon stick, broken
finely grated zest of ½ orange
2 tablespoons shelled hemp seeds (optional)

1. Mix the pudding rice and brown rice in a saucepan with 650ml of the rice milk. Crush the cardamom pods lightly in a pestle and mortar or with the side of a knife to release their flavour. Stir into the rice mixture and add the cinnamon and orange zest.

2. Cook on the hob over a low heat for around 30 minutes, or until the rice is soft and the milk rich and creamy. Stir frequently towards the end of the cooking time and add more rice milk if the pudding thickens too much.

3. Serve warm. Alternatively, remove the cinnamon and divide the rice between dessert dishes or ramekins. Cover and leave to cool for 30 minutes, then chill in the fridge for 3–4 hours or until set. When cold, turn out on to small plates before sprinkling with shelled hemp seeds to serve.

Healthy treats

>> Dates rolled in carob powder

>> Fruit and nut truffles (whiz dried fruit and nuts together in the food processor and shape into balls, then roll in sesame seeds or carob powder)

>> Crunchy veggie crisps: thinly slice 1 sweet potato, 1 beet and 1 parsnip. Place in an oiled baking dish and shake over some herbal seasoning and cook for 10–15 minutes at 200°C/gas mark 6.

>> Dried fruit: dates, apricots, goji berries, figs, prunes, raisins, currants, blueberries, hunza apricots

>> Cacao nibs

>> Fruit smoothies

>> Sprouted wheat bread with raisins

>> Fruit and nut bars. Make sure they are sugar and additive free.

BOOT CAMP
WORKSHEETS

DAY 1

DECLARATION OF INTENT:

. . . .

. . . .

. . . .

. . . .

. . . .

. . . .

FOOD AND MY EMOTIONS:

. . . .

. . . .

. . . .

. . . .

. . . .

. . . .

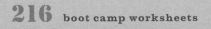

DAY 1

WEIGHT:

. . . .

MEASUREMENTS

WAIST:

. . . .

BUST:

. . . .

HIPS:

. . . .

THIGHS:

. . . .

DRESS/TROUSER SIZE:

. . . .

BMI:

. . . .

HEALTH QUIZ SCORE:

. . . .

DAY 2

PRIORITY ACTIONS (EATING):

. . . .

. . . .

. . . .

. . . .

. . . .

. . . .

PRIORITY ACTIONS (LIFESTYLE):

. . . .

. . . .

. . . .

. . . .

. . . .

. . . .

DAY 2
FOOD DIARY

TIME

BREAKFAST [   ]
....
HOW I FEEL:

SNACK [   ]
....
HOW I FEEL:

LUNCH [   ]
....
HOW I FEEL:

SNACK [   ]
....
HOW I FEEL:

DINNER [   ]
....
HOW I FEEL:

SNACK [   ]
....
HOW I FEEL:

DAY 3
MEAL PLANNER

MONDAY	TUESDAY	WEDNESDAY	THURSDAY
Breakfast	Breakfast	Breakfast	Breakfast
Snack	Snack	Snack	Snack
Lunch	Lunch	Lunch	Lunch
Snack	Snack	Snack	Snack
Dinner	Dinner	Dinner	Dinner
Snack	Snack	Snack	Snack

DAY 3

FRIDAY	SATURDAY	SUNDAY	NOTES
Breakfast	Breakfast	Breakfast	
Snack	Snack	Snack	
Lunch	Lunch	Lunch	
Snack	Snack	Snack	
Dinner	Dinner	Dinner	
Snack	Snack	Snack	

DAY 3

GOAL SETTING

OBJECTIVE:

· ·

STEP 1:

· ·

STEP 2:

· ·

STEP 3:

· ·

DAY 3

DAILY MINI GOALS:

· ·

· ·

· ·

· ·

· ·

· ·

HEALTHY TREATS:

· ·

· ·

· ·

· ·

· ·

· ·

DAY 3
FOOD DIARY

TIME

BREAKFAST   [   ]
· ·
HOW I FEEL:

SNACK   [   ]
· ·
HOW I FEEL:

LUNCH   [   ]
· ·
HOW I FEEL:

SNACK   [   ]
· ·
HOW I FEEL:

DINNER   [   ]
· ·
HOW I FEEL:

SNACK   [   ]
· ·
HOW I FEEL:

DAY 3
NOTES

....
....
....
....
....
....
....
....
....
....
....
....

DAY 4
TIME DIARY

WHAT I DID	WHY I DID IT	TIME IT TOOK

DAY 4
MUST DO TODAY!

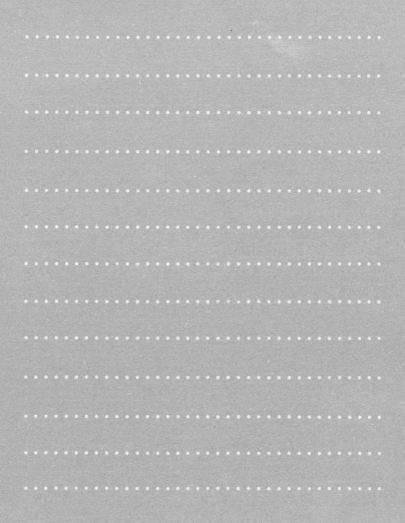

....

....

....

....

....

....

....

....

....

....

....

DAY 4
FOOD DIARY

	TIME
BREAKFAST	[ ]

HOW I FEEL:

SNACK	[ ]

HOW I FEEL:

LUNCH	[ ]

HOW I FEEL:

SNACK	[ ]

HOW I FEEL:

DINNER	[ ]

HOW I FEEL:

SNACK	[ ]

HOW I FEEL:

DAY 4
NOTES

DAY 5

EXCUSE:

· ·

· ·

· ·

· ·

**REASONS WHY THIS IS
SIMPLY NOT JUSTIFIED:**

· ·

· ·

· ·

· ·

POSITIVE STATEMENT:

· ·

· ·

· ·

· ·

DAY 5
FOOD DIARY

TIME

BREAKFAST .... [   ]

HOW I FEEL:

SNACK .... [   ]

HOW I FEEL:

LUNCH .... [   ]

HOW I FEEL:

SNACK .... [   ]

HOW I FEEL:

DINNER .... [   ]

HOW I FEEL:

SNACK .... [   ]

HOW I FEEL:

DAY 6
PROGRESS CHECKLIST

01 WHAT HAVE YOU FOUND EASIEST SO FAR ABOUT THE BOOT CAMP?

02 WHAT HAS SEEMED HARDEST?

03 WHAT NEW FOODS HAVE YOU MOST ENJOYED?

04 HAVE YOU FELT HUNGRY OR HAD CRAVINGS FOR CERTAIN FOODS AT ANY POINT?

05 HOW HAVE YOU FELT BEFORE AND AFTER EXERCISING?

06 HAVE YOU HAD ANY SLIPS, AND NOT STUCK TO THE BOOT CAMP? IF SO, WHEN, AND WHY?

07 HAVE ANY OF THE TASKS BEEN PARTICULARLY DIFFICULT FOR YOU?

08 IS YOUR LOG BOOK AN HONEST RECOLLECTION OF HOW THE PAST 5 DAYS HAVE BEEN, OR HAVE YOU MISSED ANYTHING OUT?

09 WHEN HAVE YOU FELT MOST SAD OR FRUSTRATED?

10 WHEN HAVE YOU FELT YOUR MOST HAPPY AND OPTIMISTIC?

PATTERNS:

. . . .

. . . .

. . . .

DAY 6
PERSONAL REPORT

THE POSITIVES:

01
. . . .

02
. . . .

03
. . . .

THE AREAS TO WORK ON:

01
. . . .

02
. . . .

03
. . . .

DAY 6
FOOD DIARY

TIME

BREAKFAST   [   ]
· ·
HOW I FEEL:

SNACK   [   ]
· ·
HOW I FEEL:

LUNCH   [   ]
· ·
HOW I FEEL:

SNACK   [   ]
· ·
HOW I FEEL:

DINNER   [   ]
· ·
HOW I FEEL:

SNACK   [   ]
· ·
HOW I FEEL:

DAY 6
NOTES

DAY 7

DEALING WITH DE-MOTIVATORS:

. . . .

. . . .

. . . .

. . . .

. . . .

. . . .

. . . .

. . . .

. . . .

. . . .

. . . .

. . . .

DAY 7
FOOD DIARY

TIME

BREAKFAST .... [   ]

HOW I FEEL:

SNACK .... [   ]

HOW I FEEL:

LUNCH .... [   ]

HOW I FEEL:

SNACK .... [   ]

HOW I FEEL:

DINNER .... [   ]

HOW I FEEL:

SNACK .... [   ]

HOW I FEEL:

DAY 8

POSITIVE AFFIRMATIONS:

....

....

....

....

....

....

....

....

....

....

....

....

DAY 8
FOOD DIARY

TIME

BREAKFAST   [   ]
···
HOW I FEEL:

SNACK   [   ]
···
HOW I FEEL:

LUNCH   [   ]
···
HOW I FEEL:

SNACK   [   ]
···
HOW I FEEL:

DINNER   [   ]
···
HOW I FEEL:

SNACK   [   ]
···
HOW I FEEL:

DAY 9
THE PIE OF LIFE

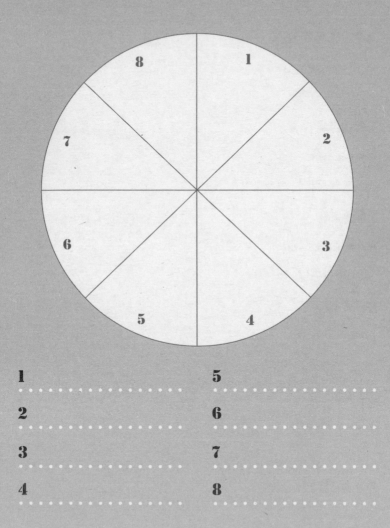

1 ....

2 ....

3 ....

4 ....

5 ....

6 ....

7 ....

8 ....

DAY 9
FOOD DIARY

TIME

BREAKFAST [ ]
·······································
HOW I FEEL:

SNACK [ ]
·······································
HOW I FEEL:

LUNCH [ ]
·······································
HOW I FEEL:

SNACK [ ]
·······································
HOW I FEEL:

DINNER [ ]
·······································
HOW I FEEL:

SNACK [ ]
·······································
HOW I FEEL:

DAY 10
FOOD DIARY

TIME

BREAKFAST   [   ]
· ·
HOW I FEEL:

SNACK   [   ]
· ·
HOW I FEEL:

LUNCH   [   ]
· ·
HOW I FEEL:

SNACK   [   ]
· ·
HOW I FEEL:

DINNER   [   ]
· ·
HOW I FEEL:

SNACK   [   ]
· ·
HOW I FEEL:

DAY 10
NOTES

....

....

....

....

....

....

....

....

....

....

....

DAY 11

DAILY ROUTINE CHANGES:

01
....

02
....

03
....

FUN ACTIVITIES:

01
....

02
....

03
....

DAY 11
FOOD DIARY

TIME

BREAKFAST   [   ]
· ·
HOW I FEEL:

SNACK   [   ]
· ·
HOW I FEEL:

LUNCH   [   ]
· ·
HOW I FEEL:

SNACK   [   ]
· ·
HOW I FEEL:

DINNER   [   ]
· ·
HOW I FEEL:

SNACK   [   ]
· ·
HOW I FEEL:

DAY 12

SHOPPING CONSCIOUSLY:

....

....

....

....

....

....

....

....

....

....

....

....

DAY 12
FOOD DIARY

TIME

BREAKFAST [ ]
· ·
HOW I FEEL:

SNACK [ ]
· ·
HOW I FEEL:

LUNCH [ ]
· ·
HOW I FEEL:

SNACK [ ]
· ·
HOW I FEEL:

DINNER [ ]
· ·
HOW I FEEL:

SNACK [ ]
· ·
HOW I FEEL:

DAY 13
FOOD DIARY

TIME

BREAKFAST [   ]

HOW I FEEL:

SNACK [   ]

HOW I FEEL:

LUNCH [   ]

HOW I FEEL:

SNACK [   ]

HOW I FEEL:

DINNER [   ]

HOW I FEEL:

SNACK [   ]

HOW I FEEL:

DAY 13
NOTES

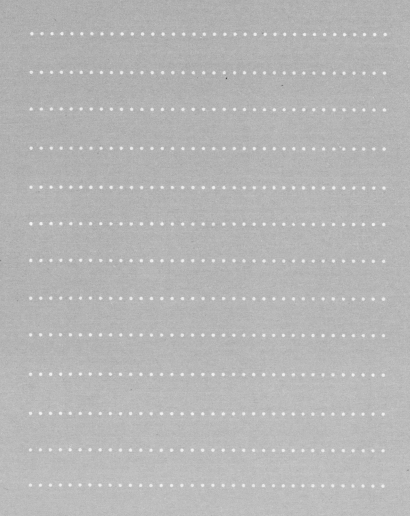

DAY 14

HEALTH QUIZ SCORE:

· ·

POSITIVE REALIZATIONS:

· ·

· ·

· ·

· ·

· ·

· ·

· ·

· ·

· ·

· ·

DAY 14
DECLARATION OF INTENT

....
....
....
....
....
....
....
....
....
....
....
....

ACKNOWLEDGEMENTS

A big Boot Camp thank you to all my Boot Campers.
Keep Boot Camping!

A massive thank you to Howard for your help and tremendous
support for this Boot Camp. To Dawn too for your inspiration,
dedication and tenacity. Deep gratitude to Sue also. So many
thanks to Hannah. Warm wishes to Josie.

Many thanks to Kate Adams at Penguin for your insight
and unwavering determination to help get out my message
that each and every one of us should do as much as we can
to take back the reins of our health and lifestyle. Thanks
so much to Sarah and Bethan too. And big hugs all round
to Louise, Tom and Katy for all that you do.

Appreciation to Nicola, Jonny and Luigi.

Many thanks to Martin and Relton for the behind-the-
scenes support of spreading the word and advancing my
healthy-living mission, so that together we may improve
the lives of people everywhere.

WWW.GILLIANMCKEITH.INFO

Empowering people to improve their lives through information, food and lifestyle.

Join the club at:
www.gillianmckeithclub.com
As a member, you will have access to a wide range of tools, resources and features that will support you further. Take control of your life.

The Gillian McKeith Club includes:

- » Gillian's Boot Camp
- » Personal Health Profile
- » Club News
- » Club Forum
- » Research Centre
- » Nutrition Clinic
- » Live Chats with Gillian
- » Weekly Top Tips
- » Weekly Meal Plans
- » Meal Ideas and Recipes
- » Newsletter
- » And more!

GILLIAN MCKEITH'S BOOT CAMP WALKING WORKOUTS

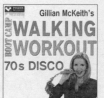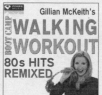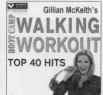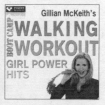

A range of 30-minute audio workouts you can do anywhere at any time. Choose your workout from today's top 40 hits, 70s disco or 80s classics, with more coming soon. Just download, play and get moving – walking, jogging, stretching, dancing!

Each audio download features Gillian's expert instruction to great music. Download now to your iPod or MP3 player. Available at **iTunes**®, **www.tescodigital.com** (search under Gillian McKeith) or **www.gillianmckeith.info**.

>> **An easy-to-download workout programme that fits in with any lifestyle.**

>> **Get maximum results in minimum time.**

>> **Look great and keep fit, the Gillian McKeith Way!**

Gillian says, 'Walking is the best exercise in the world. It's low impact, easy to do, and you can easily fit it into your lifestyle. So no excuses! Join me today, let's walk and workout together. And I'll even give you a few motivational tips along the way.'

GILLIAN MCKEITH BECOMES YOUR TRAINER TO WALK AND WORKOUT WITH!

live more

If you would like to receive more information on Healthy Penguin titles, authors, special offers, events and giveaways, please email HealthyPenguin@uk.penguingroup.com